LISTENING TO THE VOICES
OF LONG-TERM CARE

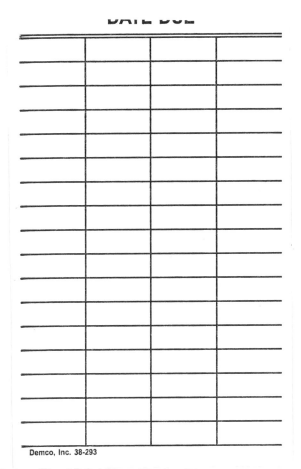
Lanham · Boulder · New York · Toronto · Plymouth, UK

Copyright © 2007 by
University Press of America,® Inc.
4501 Forbes Boulevard
Suite 200
Lanham, Maryland 20706
UPA Acquisitions Department (301) 459-3366

Estover Road
Plymouth PL6 7PY
United Kingdom

Library of Congress Control Number: 2007929172
ISBN-13: 978-0-7618-3815-9 (clothbound : alk. paper)
ISBN-10: 0-7618-3815-5 (clothbound : alk. paper)
ISBN-13: 978-0-7618-3816-6 (paperback : alk. paper)
ISBN-10: 0-7618-3816-3 (paperback : alk. paper)

Table of Contents

LIST OF TABLES

LIST OF FIGURES

Preface

The need for this book was recognized when former students, current long-term care administrators, returned to campus stating that they were not prepared for the intensity of the human interactions and personal dilemmas they were encountering in their work. In reviewing textbooks from the field, I did find many long-term care books available. However, most of them provided either intensive descriptions of long-term care services and polices or dealt with in-depth nursing home management; none of them addressed the human complexities involved in the design and delivery of these services. This book addresses the human quality of long-term care services and prepares readers to provide more sensitive, responsive, assistance to the individuals they serve. It provides insight into the needs of primary clients (aging individuals and their families) while recognizing the unique characteristics of core staff (nursing assistants and nurses), and examines the connections between the two.

There are several unique characteristics of this book. First, it is about individuals who are either working in or using long-term care services. Their voices are heard through reports from personal interviews, focus groups, surveys, and, at times undercover observations. Many different researchers contributed their studies, and to my knowledge, they have never been collated in such a manner. This gathering of information provides a truly rich, intimate portrait of the essential aspects of long term care. Other unique characteristics include:

- All chapters provide examples of long-term care from home care agencies and assisted-living facilities as well as from nursing homes. Perspectives of individuals just beginning to use services as well as the views of those who have received services for many years are presented. The continuum of long-term care follows with chapters outlining the voices of staff members including those who work in clients' homes and those working elsewhere in long-term care organizations.

- Discussion questions are provided at the end of each chapter. These thought provoking questions are designed to be useful either as student homework or as topics for group discussions. The questions are presented in such a way as to be interesting for use after reading the book when comparing voices would provide a deepening of understanding.

- This book can effectively be used with both undergraduate and graduate students in related courses. Graduate students (masters or doctoral level) may review primary studies referenced at the end of the book, while undergraduate students may directly delve into the described findings. Questions at the end of each chapter provide students an opportunity to reflect on their understanding of the reading as they challenge themselves by searching for effective responses that move long-term care to a higher level of sensitivity and care.

Chapter one opens with a brief description of seniors in the United States. It describes where they live and their functional characteristics, and serves as an introduction for students new to long-term care issues. The book then really opens with chapter two. This chapter begins with descriptions of the needs and experiences of aging individuals and their families as they consider accessing services and as they receive services in their homes, communities, or nursing homes. Satisfactions and dissatisfactions, as well as fears and concerns, are heard. In this chapter, aging persons with different degrees of need are presented. The first seniors considered are living in their own homes in the community, but talk about the possibility of one day using long-term care services. The next group of seniors heard live in their homes, but use the services of a home care worker for assistance. The level and extent of home care varies from one day a week to everyday; note that all have definite preferences about the services they receive. Finally, we hear from seniors who have lost their homes and who are adjusting to congregate living in assisted-living facilities or nursing homes. Seniors in their early moments of using these services—and those who have lived many years with these services—are represented. This chapter describes seniors' preferences for workers and specific services or activities from their own perspectives, expressed in their own voices.

Chapter three is one of the longest chapters as it provides reflections from frontline staff; these staff members provide nearly 80% of the care and daily services on which seniors depend. Nationwide, there are at least 2 million frontline workers; nearly 90 % of them are women. Their wages are very low, even when compared with other low-wage jobs, and many live paycheck to paycheck and hold multiple jobs to make ends meet. Despite the fact that these assistants provide the majority of care within long-term care organizations, their voices and attitudes are difficult to reveal. In order to listen to their voices, some researchers interviewed them; others worked alongside them, closely observing their work and treatment within the organizations in which they worked.

Chapter four provides descriptions of a typical day experienced by nursing home, assisted-living, and home care nurses. It includes details of the daily functions that these nurses regularly perform in long-term care settings. Some activities, such as teaching, are performed more frequently by home care nurses, while other activities, such as supervising, are performed more frequently by assisted-living and nursing home nurses. Nurses' satisfactions and reasons for working in long-term care organizations are reported. Last, nurses' challenges and reasons for burnout are examined.

The administrative voices comprise chapter five and come from the senior managers of nursing homes, home care agencies, and assisted-living facilities. They include both CEOs and senior nurse administrators who are often called directors of nursing services. This chapter considers both the collective and individual voices of administrators identified by organizational responsibility. The chapter begins by describing the typical functions of long-term care administrators; each administrative position has a core of fundamental tasks and responsibilities that have been identified by specific job analysis studies. Next, administrators' personal and professional values are presented. The chapter ends with administrators' major challenges and dissatisfactions. As the chapter will reveal, an increasing number of long-term care administrators are not renewing their administrative licenses; possible reasons for this finding are explored.

The purpose of chapter six is to identify the similarities and differences of the major stakeholders within long-term care systems. Daily activities, as well as personal and professional values, are reviewed for each stakeholder. These perspectives are compared to identify shared aims and common needs. In listening to the lists of administrators' daily tasks, it is clear that their work is often more than one individual can achieve without support, and systemic challenges exist. However, it is just as clear that with more communication, with real listening and understanding among team members, better care for seniors is possible.

Chapter seven, the closing chapter, presents successful programs and strategies that address concerns heard from both seniors and caregivers; many excellent programs are examined. Successful client programs include programs that focus on seniors' health and on their functional and psychosocial needs. It is hoped that this final chapter will take students to a starting point for developing new programs that are responsive to both clients and staff. This chapter helps students put the range of voices within a working perspective and assists them in focusing on ensuring that clients control most aspects of their own care. Successful staff programs are those that promote staff dignity, professional values, and growth with the intention of promoting job satisfaction and retention. The beginning of this chapter illustrates how programs and strategies must be viewed as organizational packages and not as stand-alone programs, while the final section describes program components addressing the special needs of both clients and staff.

In conclusion, the title of this book includes the term "listening," and there is an intended purpose for that. Numerous studies confirm that listening is one of the most critical skills for leadership success. In fact, skillful listening is the foundation for all the popular and effective leadership training programs such as those of Steven Covey, Daniel Goleman, and Peter Drucker. While listening is a means of professional growth, it is also a tool for personal enlightenment. As you listen to the voices within this book, there should be two areas of focus: 1) listening to and recognizing yourself in relation to these voices and 2) listening and responding to the concerns and cries of others. As you read, I invite you to listen with care and compassion to the voice within yourself as well as to the voices of others that are here presented.

JRB

Acknowledgments

This book could not have been written without the generous help of my parents. For many summers they lovingly took care of my daughter, Jackie, while I "worked on the book." I gladly owe them a debt of thanks. My friend and editor, Aeron Hicks, provided the final support I needed during the last months of finishing this book. I thank her for her encouragement and fine skills as a writer, as well as for our wonderful friendship.

My students at the University of South Dakota have been the first audience for many of these chapters. I thank them for their patient reading and thoughtful comments. More than this, I also thank them for their interest and commitment to the long-term care field. I have no doubt they will make this world a better place through their insights and understanding.

Many of my colleagues and graduate students have given valuable feedback and helped the manuscript make its way to completion. I offer my thanks to Bill Ross, Jenny Dewald, Mike Gillispie, and Mike Myers, who reviewed materials and provided their support.

Finally, I thank all the researchers referenced in this book. Their dedication and commitment to hearing the true voices within long-term care constantly amazed me. Their creativity, patience, and meticulous work are the hidden voices behind this book. I hope that they will find my interpretation of their findings satisfactory. Of course, any errors or gaps in this work are only to be attributed to me.

JRB

❦

CHAPTER 1

THE LONG-TERM CARE SYSTEM AND OUR SENIORS

"Listening is the act of ac-
knowledging the unique
value of the thoughts and
opinions of others." [1]

It is becoming more and more evident that the rapidly expanding long-term care industry will only continue to grow as a greater percentage of Americans age and need more health care services. However, perhaps not as evident are the looming challenges that long-term care organizations face. As the Baby Boomers age, Americans are demanding more from their health care services than ever before, and they want organizations that are sensitive and alert to their needs and desires as they grow older.

The health care workers who provide the fundamental day-to-day services that sustain seniors are now recognized as one of the industry's greatest concerns. Personal care assistants, as well as professional nurses, have some of the highest employee turnover rates of those in any industry. This is not only a managerial challenge, but a service one as well. Seniors need consistent care from individuals who know them and their needs. Further contributing to this industry's stresses, an increasing number of administrators are not renewing their licenses, and there is a real and growing need for dedicated executives to provide leadership in long-term care organizations.

Success in this field starts with administrators who appreciate the challenges seniors face as their health declines and as they manage the last phases of their lives. Just as important to success is an understanding of the roles and characteristics of the various staff members who provide care and nurturing to those they serve. By listening to, reflecting upon, and then responding to the various voices within long-term care organizations, leaders can begin to provide the kind of exceptional services that today's and tomorrow's seniors will both need and expect.

This book presents the perspectives of seniors and practitioners in long-term care organizations. Their voices clarify and force us to consider the complex challenges this industry faces. Chapter Two of this text presents an overview of seniors' thoughts and concerns as they make often heart-rending decisions when recognizing and then accepting their need for new long-term care services. This information provides an illuminating backdrop for the voices presented in the following chapters. Chapters Three through Six focus on the difficulties and concerns of the industry's workforce: personal care assistants, nurses, and administrators.

An Overview of Seniors Today

A senior is defined as anyone age 65 or older. In the United States, seniors are a rapidly growing and heterogeneous population. Currently about 12% of the general population are seniors, but this percentage is increasing quickly. It is projected that by 2030, the senior population will be double that of 2000, reaching about 72 million. After 2030, the ratio of seniors to the general population is predicted to stabilize with seniors comprising about 20% of that population. Currently about 7% of seniors are age 65 to 74 (the "young old"), 4% are age 75 to 84 (the "middle old"), and 2% are 85 and older (the "oldest old"). As Figure 1.1 reveals, while the whole senior population will grow, the oldest old group is expected to increase the most rapidly. In 2000 there were 4.2 million seniors age 85 and older. In 2010 there are expected to be almost 10 million, and by 2050, about 21 million.[2]

Figure 1.1 Projected Growth of Aging Population

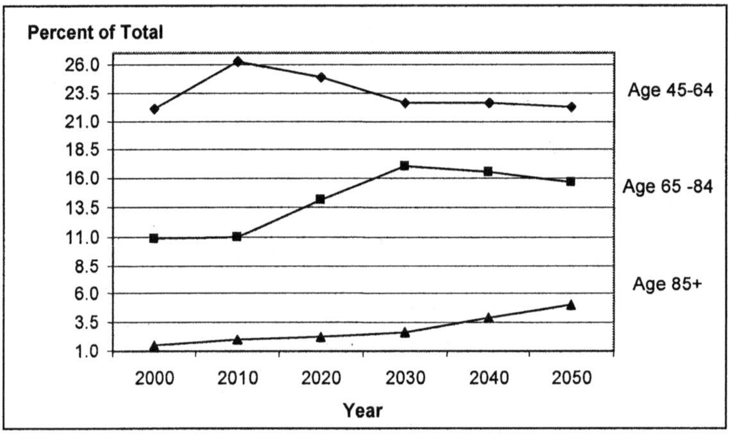

Source: U.S. Census Bureau, 2004, U.S. Interim Projections by Age, Sex, Race, and Hispanic Origin

Geographical Distribution

Seniors are not evenly distributed throughout the United States. The states with the most seniors are the most heavily populated states such as California, New York, and Florida. However, as Table 1.1 illustrates, states with the largest proportions of older people are not typically those with the greatest numbers of seniors. The three states with the highest proportions of seniors are Florida, Pennsylvania, and West Virginia with 17.6%, 15.6%, and 15.3 %, respectively. In twenty states, seniors make up between 13% and 15% of the populations, and the populations of five states include less than 10% of seniors. [3]

The aging population within communities is concentrated in specific Midwestern and Southern states. There are 3,141 counties in the United States, and in 331 of them, more than 20% of the population is 65 or older. Of these, the

100 counties with the largest percentages of seniors are in the Midwest and South. The Midwestern states with counties consisting of 20% or more seniors are Kansas (16 counties); North Dakota (15 counties), and Nebraska (11 counties).The Southern states with high proportions of seniors (20 % or more) are Florida (15 counties) and Texas (12 counties). The states experiencing the largest growth in senior population are located primarily in the West and the South. Furthermore, this growth is most rapid among the oldest segment of seniors, those with the greatest number of medical and functional challenges.[4]

Household arrangements are, of course, very significant factors in seniors' lives. Most seniors live in the community in single family homes with about 8% living in housing specially constructed for them; included are retirement communities and assisted-living facilities. Almost half of seniors live with a spouse and an average of nearly 28% live alone (see Figure 1.2). Less than 15% live with a relative other than a spouse and 2% live with non-relatives. The probability of living alone increases with age and by gender. Nearly 67% of seniors age 85 or older live alone with the majority of these older seniors being women.[5]

Table 1.1 Senior Population by State: 2000

Rank	Population 65 and over		Percent 65 and over	
	State	Number	State	Percent
1	California	3,595,658	Florida	17.6
2	Florida	2,807,597	Pennsylvania	15.6
3	New York	2,448,352	West Virginia	15.3
4	Texas	2,072,532	Iowa	14.9
5	Pennsylvania	1,919,165	North Dakota	14.7
6	Ohio	1,507,757	Rhode Island	14.5
7	Illinois	1,500,025	Maine	14.4
8	Michigan	1,219,018	South Dakota	14.3
9	New Jersey	1,113,136	Arkansas	14.0
10	North Carolina	969,048	Connecticut	13.8
11	Massachusetts	860,162	Nebraska	13.6
12	Virginia	792,333	Massachusetts	13.5
13	Georgia	785,275	Missouri	13.5
14	Missouri	755,379	Montana	13.4
15	Indiana	752,831	Ohio	13.3
16	Tennessee	703,311	Hawaii	13.3
17	Wisconsin	702,553	Kansas	13.3
18	Arizona	667,839	New Jersey	13.2
19	Washington	662,148	Oklahoma	13.2
20	Maryland	599,307	Wisconsin	13.1
21	Minnesota	594,266	Alabama	13.0
22	Alabama	579,798	Arizona	13.0
23	Louisiana	516,929	Delaware	13.0
24	Kentucky	504,793	New York	12.9
25	South Carolina	485,333	Oregon	12.8
26	Connecticut	470,183	Vermont	12.7
27	Oklahoma	455,950	Kentucky	12.5

28	Oregon	438,177	Indiana	12.4
29	Iowa	436,213	Tennessee	12.4
30	Colorado	416,073	Michigan	12.3
31	Arkansas	374,019	District of Columbia	12.2
32	Kansas	356,229	South Carolina	12.1
33	Mississippi	343,523	Minnesota	12.1
34	West Virginia	276,895	Illinois	12.1
35	Nebraska	232,195	Mississippi	12.1
36	Nevada	218,929	North Carolina	12.0
37	New Mexico	212,225	New Hampshire	12.0
38	Utah	190,222	Wyoming	11.7
39	Maine	183,402	New Mexico	11.7
40	Hawaii	160,601	Louisiana	11.6
41	Rhode Island	152,402	Maryland	11.3
42	New Hampshire	147,970	Idaho	11.3
43	Idaho	145,916	Washington	11.2
44	Montana	120,949	Virginia	11.2
45	South Dakota	108,131	Nevada	11.0
46	Delaware	101,726	California	10.6
47	North Dakota	94,478	Texas	9.9
48	Vermont	77,510	Colorado	9.7
49	District of Columbia	69,898	Georgia	9.6
50	Wyoming	57,693	Utah	8.5
51	Alaska	35,699	Alaska	5.7

Source: U.S. Census Bureau, 2001

Figure 1.2 Percent of Population Aged 65 and Over Living Alone: 1980-2003

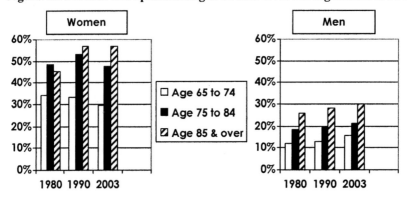

Source: U.S. Census Bureau, Current Population Survey, Annual Social and Economic Supplement, 2004

Socioeconomic Status

Historically, seniors have seen an uneven climb in their household incomes. Today, the median household income for seniors is lower than the median income for younger households, but it is considerably more than it was a decade ago. The census data reveal that household income typically increases with age until age 45 to 54, when it starts to decline.[6] Seniors' personal income comes primarily from four sources: Social Security, earnings, pensions, and asset income with Social Security providing the largest share. The amount of money a senior receives from Social Security varies by earning history, as well as by the age at which he or she started drawing on it. A senior with relatively high past earnings will receive more Social Security than one with a history of lower earnings. Likewise, seniors who wait to draw their Social Security will receive more money per payout than seniors who begin drawing their Social Security at earlier ages (e.g., age 62 versus age 70). As can be imagined, senior women receive considerably less Social Security income than do senior men.

A more realistic and complete picture of seniors' economic status emerges when we examine personal wealth figured in terms of median net worth. This figure is composed of all personal assets, such as equity in one's home, personal savings, and stocks and bonds. At first glance, seniors appear to be much better off than the general population. In 2000, the median net worth of households in the U.S. was $55,000, while for seniors, it was $108,885. However, the personal wealth of seniors has a skewed distribution with nearly two thirds of seniors in the lowest quintiles and just 17% in the upper quintiles.[7]

Currently, 10.2% of seniors live below the poverty line. The percentage of young people (under age 18) living below the poverty line is 17.6%, while about 11% of people aged 18 to 64 live in poverty.[8] However, despite seniors' relatively low poverty rates, this population contains pockets of seniors who are living in extreme poverty. Senior women are more likely to live in poverty than are senior men (2.5% and 7.3%, respectively), and older seniors are more likely to be poor than younger seniors. Seniors aged 65 to 74 have a poverty rate of 9%, compared with nearly 12% for seniors 75 and older. Living alone and ethnicity are other predictors of poverty; older seniors who live alone experience the highest rates. Over 17% of older White women living alone have incomes below the poverty level, while nearly 40% of Black and Hispanic women living alone survive on below-poverty-level incomes.[9]

Seniors' employment status is related to their economic status in multiple ways. Certainly, seniors have a lower employment rate than the general population. In 2003, nearly 66% of men and 55% of women age 55 to 64 were employed, compared with nearly 12 % of men and 6% of women age 70 and older. However, as Table 1.2 reveals many seniors work part time, and the proportion of older workers who work part time increases with age for both men and women. Nearly 50% of women and just over 60% of men 70 or older work only part-time.[10]

Table 1.2 Employment Status and Age: 2003

Gender and Age	Total	Employed Total	Employed Percent of population	Percent Employed Full-time	Percent Employed Part-time
Men					
55 to 64	13,305	8,733	65.6	89.6	10.4
65 to 69	4,449	1,397	31.4	65.2	34.8
70 and over	10,047	1,188	11.8	53.3	46.7
Women					
55 to 64	14,423	7,866	54.5	76.1	23.9
65 to 69	5,142	1,119	21.8	50.7	49.3
70 and over	14,616	905	6.2	39.0	60.9

Source: Bureau of Labor Statistics, 2004a

Older men are more likely than older women to be married (71% versus 41%). The proportion of married seniors decreases for both men and women as they age, but for women, the decrease is much steeper. Only 34% of women age 75 to 84 and only 13% of women age 85 and older are married. Similarly, widowhood is much more common among older women than older men. Women 65 and older are three times as likely as men of the same age to be widowed (44% versus 14%).[11]

Education attainment also varies among senior subgroups. In 2003, 72% of seniors held at least a high school diploma, and 13% had earned at least a bachelor's degree. Senior women are as likely as senior men to have a high school diploma; however, while 23% of senior men have a bachelor's degree, only 13% of senior women do.[12]

Compared to younger American populations, today's seniors are not very ethnically diverse. Non-Hispanic White individuals account for nearly 83% of all seniors. Blacks, Hispanics, and Asians account for 8%, 6%, and 3%, respectively. Black, Hispanic, and Asian seniors face different challenges, including decreased average life expectancy. White females born in 2000 had a life expectancy of 80 years, while Black females born the same year could expect to live about 75 years.[13] These ethnic differences in life expectancy are slowly changing as the gap in longevity between ethnicities narrows. Living arrangements also differ by ethnicity. In 2003, older Black, Asian, and Hispanic women were more likely than Non-Hispanic White women to live with relatives. Finally, senior education attainment also differs by ethnicity. In 2003, 76% of White seniors, 70% of Asians, 52% of Blacks, and 35% of Hispanics had completed high school.

Health and Functional Status of Seniors

People today are living longer and healthier lives than ever before; in 2000, the average life expectancy in the United States was nearly 77 years, up from only 47 years in 1900.[14] Generally, women have longer life expectancies than men; this is true for both Black and White women. However, this gender gap has declined in recent years due to an increase in lung cancer mortality among women and declines in heart disease in both genders. There are also racial differences in life expectancy; in 2000, the White population had a life expectancy of 77.4 years, while the Black population had a life expectancy of only 71.7 years. These racial differences grow smaller and actually reverse at older ages. Table 1.3 shows the racial gap in life expectancy in five-year increments. At age 85 and above, the Black/White differences in life expectancy fall to nearly zero, and at ages older than 85, Black seniors have longer life expectancies than their White counterparts.[15]

Table 1.3 Life Expectancy by Sex and Race: 2000

Age	*Male*			*Female*		
	White	Black	Difference (Black minus White)	White	Black	Difference (Black minus White)
0	74.8	68.2	-6.6	80.0	74.9	-5.1
65	16.3	14.5	-1.8	19.2	17.4	-1.8
70	13.0	11.7	-1.3	15.5	14.1	-1.4
75	10.1	9.4	-0.7	12.1	11.2	-0.9
80	7.6	7.3	-0.3	9.1	8.6	-0.5
85	5.5	5.7	0.2	6.6	6.5	-0.1
90	4.0	4.5	0.5	4.7	4.8	0.1
95	2.9	3.6	0.7	3.3	3.6	0.3
100	2.2	2.9	0.7	2.4	2.7	0.3

Source: National Center for Health Statistics, 2002

Healthy aging involves not only a long life free of disease, but high physical and mental functioning, significant engagement with friends, and engagement in productive activities.[16] It is evident that chronic diseases, physical disabilities, and mental conditions can severely impact a senior's health. Yet chronic diseases and disabilities are a part of most seniors' lives; about 80% of seniors have been diagnosed with at least one chronic illness, and 50% with at least two.[17]

A chronic disease is defined as an illness that persists for three months or more. These diseases generally cannot be prevented by vaccines or cured by medication, and they are rarely cured completely.[18] Although genetics contribute significantly to the development of chronic diseases, we would do well to remember that negative personal behaviors such as tobacco use, lack of physical activity, and poor eating habits also contribute. Chronic diseases are leading causes of disability and economic burden. The most common chronic diseases among seniors are arthritis, hypertension, heart disease, diabetes, and respiratory disorders. Although both genders suffer from these diseases, older women are more likely to suffer from hypertension and arthritis, while older men are more likely to suffer from heart disease.[19] Figure 1.3 reveals gender differences for common chronic diseases.

Figure 1.3 Common Chronic Diseases among Seniors

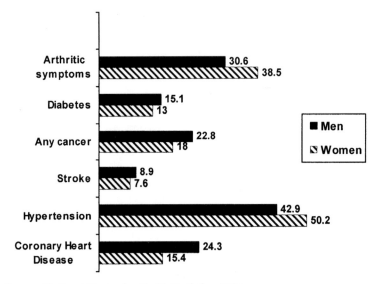

Source: National Center for Health Statistics, 2004

Chronic diseases are often related to disabilities, which are commonly defined in terms of degrees of difficulty in performing activities of daily living (ADL). There are eleven functions officially recognized as ADL; the five most basic functions are the abilities to dress, eat, ambulate (walk), go to the toilet, and take care of personal hygiene. Instrumental activities of daily living (IADL) are functions necessary to live independently in the community. The most basic IADL assessed are the abilities to shop, keep house, manage personal finances, prepare food, and get around (e.g., driving).[20]

Disabilities, of course, often lead to loss of independence. In 2000, about 42% of seniors had at least one disability. About 20% of seniors have a chronic disability, about 7% have a severe cognitive impairment, and about 30% experience mobility difficulties.[21] The number of seniors with disabilities has been declining for the last two decades. This trend is attributed to several factors, including improved medical treatment, positive behavioral changes, increased use of assistive technology, and improved socioeconomic status. Some medical treatments, such as medicines (e.g., for arthritis and hypertension), new surgeries (e.g., cataract and joint replacements), and sophisticated assistive devices (e.g., telemedicine computers and programmed wheelchairs) enable seniors to maintain their independence. Figure 1.4 shows the number of individuals with limitations caused by chronic health conditions by age group and reveals the significant number of seniors compared to younger age groups who are affected.

Figure 1.4 Individuals with Activity Limitations from Chronic Disease *

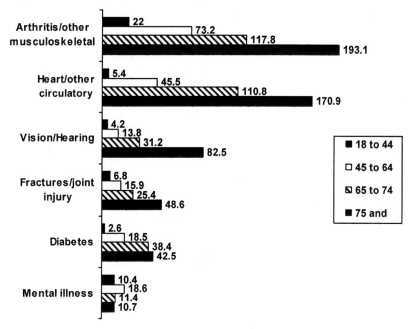

*This chart displays the number of people with limitations caused by chronic health conditions per 1,000 population 1998 to 2000).
Source: National Center for Health Statistics, 2002a, Figure 17

Sensory impairments such as loss of vision or hearing also clearly decrease seniors' independence. These impairments make seniors more prone to falling, and can lead to loss of social activities and can exacerbate depression. The most common causes of visual impairment and loss among older people are cataracts, age-related macular degeneration, glaucoma, and diabetic retinopathy. In 2000, only 0.5% of the population under age 65 faced hearing- or vision-related limitations in activities, yet over 8% of those 75 years and older experienced such limitations. Hearing loss seems more prevalent; about 33% of seniors age 75 and older and almost 50% of those aged 85 and older have hearing impairments. Worst of all, about 20% of seniors age 70 and older, experience both hearing and visual impairments. These seniors are more likely to fall, break hips, and develop hypertension, heart disease, or strokes than those who retain hearing and/or vision. For understandable reasons, they also report engaging in fewer social activities.[22]

Long-Term Care and Health Care Services

The general definition of long-term care is a combination of health care, personal care, and social services that are provided over a sustained period of time to persons who have lost some degree of functional ability.[23] Whereas health care is generally episodic and most often results in curing illness or restoring a previous state of health, long-term care helps individuals to function as well as possible for as long as possible despite their health. The boundaries between the two are admittedly blurry.

Prior to our discussion of long-term care organizations, it should be noted that while the majority of long-term care service users are seniors, not all are. Younger users typically have developmental disabilities and need some level of care all their lives, while seniors typically need care for only limited amount of time during the latter part of their lives. One of the most significant differences between younger and older long-term care recipients is that younger recipients typically are covered by Medicaid or receive payments from Supplemental Security Income (SSI) and don't seem to struggle with the same funding issues that seniors do. Approximately 43% of long-term care recipients are under 64, while 57% are 65 or over. [24]

Health Care Utilization

Office visits and hospitalizations are the health care services seniors most frequently seek, and they consistently use more health care as they age. The U.S. Census Bureau reports that 34% of those aged 65 to 74 make an average of 4 to 9 health care visits in a year, compared to 39% of those aged 75 and over. Hospitalizations also increase with age. Seniors over 65 years are hospitalized twice as often as people under 65, stay twice as long once they are admitted, and use twice as many prescription drugs during their hospiralizations.[25]

Long-Term Care Services

Long-term care is often described as a continuum of services, ranging from care brought to one's home such as home health care to community services such as adult day care, to institutional services such as those found in a skilled-nursing facility or nursing home. These services can be provided relatively infrequently (e.g., weekly) or frequently (e.g., daily), and can be offered by multiple service providers or just one. Furthermore, health care and long-term care services are often integrated because seniors with acute health care needs so often experience functional disabilities. Over the last two decades the number and variety of long-term care organizations have proliferated. This is due not only to the growing number of seniors but also to their specific demands, as well as to government restrictions on Medicare reimbursement. The organizations presented here (Table 1.4) are those most frequently used by seniors.

Table 1.4 Long-Term Care Organizations and Services

Type of Organization	Description	Distribution & Growth	Client Descriptions	Cost & Medicare/ Medicaid Coverage
Senior Centers / Senior Clubs	Community program which is focal point for information and referrals for services. Services can include: nutritional meals, recreation, social and educational services. Center open days with variety of services (social only to medical/ mixed); provides respite to caregivers. 74% associated with other organizations.	15,000 centers throughout the nation (218 centers are certified) 10 million served annually 4,000 centers (150,000 seniors) (growing; many areas have need)	Some serve relatively young, healthy seniors. 10% of clients are over age 85 and an increasing number served are recognized as "frail elderly." Family caregivers are a new client group. Average age = 72 with ¾ living with families; majority have ADL disabilities; 50% cognitively disabled.	Fees are contingent on services or programs; usually minimal; many centers have some government funding. No Medicare or Medicaid coverage www.ncoa.org $25—$100 / day (this is approximately 8 hours) Medicare may cover some, if medical care provided; some Private insurance if enough medical care provided; if state waiver, possible assistance for low-income seniors. http://www.nadsa.org
Home care & Community Services to low income individuals	Variety of services: medical, social, personal, and respite services not covered by Medicaid – often provided in home or residential group homes.	Nearly 300 programs throughout 48 states.	Wide range of clients (50% seniors, 38% MR/DD, 17% seniors disabled enough for SNF).	Eligibility varies, but often same as Medicaid or SNF. No cost to individual, but often waiting lists from 5 – 25 months. http://www.kff.org/medicaid/7345.cfm http://www.cms.hhs.gov/MedicaidStWaivProgDemoPGI/

Type of Organization	Description	Distribution & Growth	Client Descriptions	Cost & Medicare/ Medicaid Coverage
Senior Housing & Independent- Living Facilities	Apartments & shared housing with just seniors as neighbors or ILFs offering congregate meals and other services.	25,000 senior housing units	Some apartments are for 55+; others for 62+ Clients are independent, but cannot Perform home maintenance	Wide Range depending on luxury; $500 (with roommate) $1000—$4000 /month Medicare / Medicaid do not cover. http://www.helpguide .org/elder/ http://seniorhousing.org
Assisted- Living Facilities	Facility which provides rooms or apartments with meals and various personal support services, such as housekeeping, laundry, and some ADL assistance. Daily medication monitoring.	36,450 facilities Rapid growth 2000; now stable number.	Clients average age = 80, needing ADL, housekeeping, and medication assistance.	Medicare does not cover; Medicaid in some states, but very low reimbursement; often not accepted in ALFs (only 11% of clients now). Average $2,379 month (range $2000—$4,000/ month) www.alfa.org http://aspe.hhs.gov/da ltcp/reports/04alcom1 .htm www.ncal.org/about/ 2004_reg_review.pdf
Skilled- Nursing Fa- cilities	Nursing home with 24-hr RN or LPN; MD on call; traditionally hospital-like with semi- private rooms & nursing	16,000 with more in Mid- west & South (Number declining)	Average cli- ent aged 85 and older, very depend- ent on care for cognitive or severe physical dis- abilities.	Costs approx. $200/day or $74,000 /year Medicare coverage only with 3-day prior hospitalization & MD order; Medicaid cov- ers if client qualified as low income.

Type of Organization	Description	Distribution & Growth	Client Descriptions	Cost & Medicare/ Medicaid Coverage
	Station; social & rehabilita- tion services provided.			http://www.cdc.gov/n chs/hus.thm http://www2.aahsa.or g/aging_services/ http://www.nursingh omeinfo.com
CCRC Continuing Care Retire- ment Commu- nities or Life Care Communities	A campus of various hous- ing, residen- tial services, and health services.	2,240 licensed communities (598,000 seniors) Majority in FL, PA, KS, and CA	Average age = 80—85, but enter at younger age. Clients usu- ally need physical and financial re- view prior to acceptance.	Costs = entrance fee ($60,000—$400,000) & monthly charge ($1000—$4000) Medicare may cover some health care costs within CCRC; private LTC insur- ance may cover; Medicaid reim- bursements usually too low. http://www.seniorres ource.com/hasc.htm http://www.seniorhou singnet.com http://www.carf.org/

Source: Data compiled by Janet R. Buelow, 2006

Family and Friends

The primary goal of long-term care is to maintain the individual's independence and maximum functioning, and no service provider offers more of this
kind of care than seniors' families and friends, who are also known as "informal
caregivers." Nearly 80% of seniors receive care from family and friends, and
about 65% depend exclusively on such help. In fact, depending on the definition
of caregiving, it is estimated that from 20 to 50 million individuals, or about
20% of the total population, are caregivers of seniors. The typical caregiver is a
daughter, age 46, with a full time job. The average amount of care given per
week is 18 hours, and the average time assistance is provided is 4.5 years.[26]

The care informal caregivers provide ranges from activities of daily living
to daily tube feedings. Without the support of these informal caregivers, this
country would be financially overwhelmed. It is estimated that the services family caregivers provide for free are worth $257 billion a year. However, American

businesses lose between $11 billion and $29 billion each year as a result of employees caring for family members age 50 and older.[27]

Senior Centers

Senior centers play an important role for seniors and family caregivers in
many communities. These centers are often the first source of the social support
and referral information vital to seniors' continued independence. The official
definition of a senior center is "a place where older adults come together for
services and activities that reflect their experience and skills, respond to their
diverse needs and interests, enhance their dignity, support their independence,
and encourage their involvement in and with the center and the community."[28]
Senior centers, however, vary widely in the types and levels of services they
provide. Comprehensive centers typically provide nutrition, recreation, and social and educational services. Some of these comprehensive or "multipurpose"
senior centers are adding wellness centers and advanced education programs as
they serve younger constituents. However, many rural senior centers are small
with few resources, and they may only open for potlucks and card games.

The number of senior centers in the United States is estimated to be between 10,000 and 16,000 with the majority of centers receiving some government funding from the Older Americans Act (usually through state and area
aging agencies). Some centers are funded entirely by local non-profit organizations and others by national charitable organizations.[29]

There are national accreditation standards for senior centers which provide
official recognition of their quality and progress towards recognized missions.
These standards were developed by the National Institute of Senior Centers, a
unit within the National Council on Aging. Between 1998 and 2005, 120 senior
centers were officially accredited (or re-accredited five years after initial accreditation). These centers are dispersed throughout 29 states across the country.
Dr. A. Eugene Smiley, past chair of the National Institute of Senior Centers,
describes accreditation as the official mark of excellence for a senior center.[30]

Home Care Agencies

Arguably, the fastest growing type of long-term care is home health or
home care agencies. These organizations deliver a wide variety of care and services, ranging from professional nursing and physical therapies to personal assistance with activities of daily living. These services generally are available 24
hours a day, seven days a week, and may be provided by one individual or by a
team.

Home care organizations include home health agencies, homemaker agencies, staffing agencies or registries, and independent providers. Other organizations that provide home care services are agencies providing medical equipment
and pharmaceutical infusion therapies in the home. Of course, several types of
services may be provided by one organization. A home health agency is generally Medicare certified, and therefore seniors can use their Medicare or Medicare insurance to pay for services. However, with this certification come regulations. To be eligible for Medicare coverage, a senior must be homebound and

under a physician's care, requiring medically necessary skilled-nursing; physical, occupational, or speech therapies; medical social work; supervised home care assistance; or medical equipment and supplies.[31]

Homemaker agencies provide homemakers, aides, or assistants (paraprofessionals) who generally help with activities of daily living such as bathing, dressing, and housekeeping. These services are provided under some state regulations with minimum standards. Individual seniors often pay for these services; however, some government funding is available for seniors with financial need. Also, some agencies provide assistance from charitable foundations that aid seniors in their payments. A few seniors have health or long-term care insurance which pays for these services.

Staffing agencies or registries are private businesses providing nursing, homemaker, or assistant services. Some of these organizations accept health insurance for specific services, but often seniors must pay for homemaker services themselves. Pharmaceutical infusion therapy companies provide drugs, equipment, and professional support to seniors needing intravenous treatments. Durable medical equipment and supply dealers provide devices such as wheelchairs, walkers, and oxygen equipment. They typically install these products and instruct seniors in how to use them. These companies are either independent or Medicare-certified or work within certified home health care agencies.[32]

Senior Housing, Independent-Living Facilities, and Assisted-Living Facilities

There are many types of housing arrangements for seniors. Senior housing, typically consisting of age-restricted apartments, is for seniors with the fewest disabilities and health problems. These apartments generally do not include meal provisions, but often offer community rooms and a pool or wellness center.[33] Some senior apartment complexes have been built specifically for those needing income subsidies to assist them with paying their rent. These complexes have wheelchair friendly design features, and some provide supportive services, although most do not. There is a critical need to expand the number and availability of these affordable senior housing for older persons. For each federally subsidized apartment that becomes available, there are currently nine seniors on a waiting list.[34]

Independent-living facilities are apartments offering an array of basic services. The most common services are one congregate meal per day and assistance with laundry and light housekeeping. Most facilities are equipped with safety features and small basic kitchens, allowing seniors to prepare light meals for themselves. More and more facilities also provide recreational activities or at least transportation to these activities in the community. Often special services such as transportation, hair care, and group or individual shopping trips can be arranged.

Both senior housing and independent-living facilities provide places for seniors to be with others who share generational interests and who aren't severely disabled or ill. Both types of facilities often offer optional extra services for a fee, and neither type is regulated or licensed.

Assisted-living facilities (ALFs) provide apartments with an additional level of care. These facilities offer private apartments or rooms for seniors who need help with daily activities such as getting dressed, taking medications, transportation, meals, shopping, housekeeping, and laundry. ALFs are state regulated, although they are often called by different names (e.g., board and care, personal care homes), and regulations concerning staffing and client qualifications vary from state to state. All facilities must have at least one staff person available 24 hours a day with the majority of staff being assistants or unlicensed personnel. Clearly, seniors must have some degree of independence to live in Assisted-living Facilities. Assisted living is primarily private pay, although most states currently have a Medicaid Waiver so that seniors with Medicaid can utilize this service. However, reimbursement is often so low that these facilities are effectively unavailable to most low-income seniors.

Continuing Care Retirement Communities (CCRC) are housing and service systems in which seniors can age without having to relocate. CCRCs are generally comprised of senior housing and independent-living, assisted-living, and skilled-nursing facilities that are co-located on a single campus. Seniors move into the type of housing they initially need and then transfer to other facilities that provide more services as their needs increase. To live in a CCRC, the senior must usually pay an entrance fee and then make monthly payments corresponding to the level of services he or she receives.

Nursing Homes

A nursing home (or SNF, which stands for Skilled-Nursing Facility) provides a room, skilled-nursing care, and rehabilitation services. Some facilities (or ICFs, which stands for Intermediate-Care Facilities) provide services to younger individuals with special needs such as the developmentally disabled and mentally ill. The level of care provided by nursing homes has increased significantly over the past decade. Many now provide very skilled-nursing care and rehabilitation. Many seniors now use nursing homes for temporary recovery and then return to their own homes after a few months while others, of course, need nursing home services until the ends of their lives. Some of the services a nursing home provides include round-the-clock supervision and care, nursing care, personal care (assistance with activities of daily living), and medical services. They also offer various therapies (physical, occupational, and speech), as well as meals, laundry and housekeeping, and social and recreational activities.

Nationwide, only 4.3% of seniors live in nursing homes. Many of these seniors are the oldest old; of those aged 65 to 74, 1.1% live in nursing homes; of those aged 75 to 84, 4.5% live in nursing homes; and of those 85 and older, 18.2% live in nursing homes.[35] These numbers have decreased from a decade ago, and many attribute this decrease to increased alternative services for seniors such as home health care and assisted-living facilities. Throughout the country there are significant differences in the percentage of seniors utilizing nursing homes. As Figure 1.5 reveals, the Midwest has the highest percentage of seniors living in nursing homes (5.5% of all seniors and nearly 23% of seniors 85 and older), while on the West Coast only 2.7% of seniors live in nursing homes.[36]

Figure 1.5 Percentages of Seniors Living in Nursing Homes by Age and Region: 1999

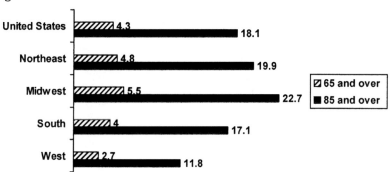

Source: National Center for Health Statistics, 2002

Conclusion

Understanding seniors' characteristics and concerns is critical to providing excellent services. Such understanding positions the health care professional to serve well and provides the insight necessary for future planning. The data clearly indicate that long-term care organizations will face increasing demands. The senior population of tomorrow will be better educated and more racially and ethnically diverse. Projections suggest that in 2030, the older population will be 72% Non-Hispanic White, 11% Hispanic, 10% Black, and 5% Asian. The gender gap in completion of a college education will narrow in the future because men and women in younger cohorts are earning college degrees at roughly the same rate. Senior work histories will be different as well. In the future older women are more likely to have worked in the paid workforce and to have their own retirement funds. Changing family structures will also impact seniors. More families are choosing not to have children, and divorce rates are increasing. Gerontologists wonder if the family support we see today will be continued for the senior parents of tomorrow.

We do not know if future seniors will live longer or if the quality of their lives will continue to improve. We also do not know if the senior disability rates that decreased during the 1980s and 1990s will continue to go down or will move back up again as more and more people reach very old age. Will healthy lifestyles and breakthroughs in public health and preventative medicine postpone the onset of disabilities and medical conditions? Increased levels of education may accompany better health, higher incomes, and more wealth, leading to higher standards of living, but we do not know the impact it will have.

Seniors face major concerns in their decisions regarding future services. These issues include the possibility of outliving their savings, managing the declining values of their homes, and paying higher costs for health care. However, more services than ever are available to seniors, and increasingly, they can demand services amenable to their preferences as well as their needs.

CR80

Discussion Questions

1.   This book defines anyone age 65 and older as a "senior" and provides three classifications of persons within this group: young old, middle old, and oldest old. What term is more appropriate for your generation's older years? Do you think your young old seniors will be the same age as today's middle old seniors (75 to 84 years)? How will age classifications differ in the next generation?

2.   Identify planning recommendations for the counties with more than 20% of their population at age 65 and older. Take into consideration the medical and functional challenges that arise as seniors age as well as the human and financial resources necessary to care for aging seniors.

3.   Seniors living alone provide a unique set of service challenges. Develop a set of criteria for identifying when it is no longer safe for someone to live alone. What services (or circumstances) would enable these individuals to live alone safely despite meeting your criteria?

4.   There are specific categories of seniors with high percentages of poverty (e.g., those living alone, Black and Hispanic women). Identify these categories of seniors and then recommend preventive measures for younger individuals who also fall within these categories so that they can decrease their probability of falling into poverty.

5.   As an employer, identify the positive and negative considerations of hiring seniors. How can employers avoid claims of age discrimination?

6.   The seniors of today are not ethnically diverse, yet the generation serving these seniors is ethnically diverse. How can cultural sensitivity be enhanced in both generations?

7.   Disabilities often lead to a senior's loss of independence; however, the number of seniors with disabilities and lost independence has been declining due to improved medical treatments, positive behavioral changes, and new assistive technologies. For each of the chronic health conditions listed in Figure 1.5, identify medical treatments, behavioral changes, and new assistive technologies that could extend seniors' independence.

8.   Approximately 43% of long-term care users are under 65 years of age. How do you think their service expectations differ from seniors who typically start using services reluctantly as their abilities decline?

9.   Seniors are hospitalized twice as often as younger adults and stay twice as long in the hospital once they are admitted. Do you think this reality can be reversed? If so, how? If not, how do you recommend that seniors pay for health care services as the senior population expands?

10. Privacy is noted as an essential preference of individuals, yet Medicare covers only semi-private rooms in the hospital and Medicaid covers semi-private rooms in a nursing home. Do you think privacy is a privilege only for those who can afford it or that Medicare and Medicaid policies should be adjusted?

11. Nearly 65% of seniors depend exclusively on care from family and friends; gerontologists wonder if the family support we see today will be continued for the senior parents of tomorrow. After all, today's families are much smaller and adult children more mobile. How and by whom will the care that is provided today by families and friends be provided to future seniors? Who do you suggest will pay for these services?

12. Many long-term care organizations describe their customers as both seniors and adult children of seniors. Describe the different expectations these two groups of consumers may have as they look into long-term care services.

13. How do the services provided in senior housing, independent-living facilities, and assisted-living facilities differ? Could a senior truly age in place in one of these facilities?

14. Seniors face major concerns regarding outliving their savings, managing the declining values of their homes, and paying the high costs of health and long-term care services. Are these concerns inevitable in life or is there a different system or model which will enable the youth of today to avoid these concerns as they age?

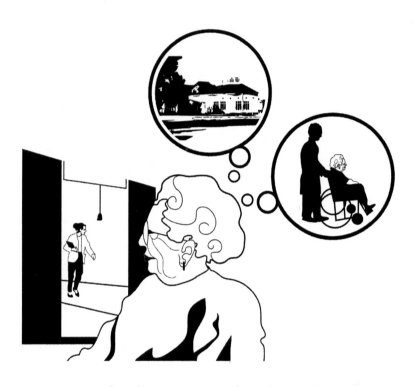

"These last years aren't going to be easy."

CHAPTER 2

VOICES OF AGING SENIORS

"In the late 1980s, I underwent a grueling medical crisis that nearly cost me my life. . . . In the crisis I experienced, I was lucky enough to find my way to a medical counselor. . . . I recall being told, 'You've been hit in a way you can't ignore. Nothing else would do it. Now you know. You are very, very sick. You might die.' So what are you going to make of that?" [1]

Long-term care services are founded on serving aging individuals as they struggle to live their final years with dignity and safety. The experiences of these individuals as they identify problems, select services, and evaluate workers compose the essential focus of this chapter. These voices cannot and do not speak for each individual senior, but they open a window on the vast array of needed care and services. It must be remembered that the voices of these seniors are influenced by personal beliefs, cultural identities, economic status, and gender as much as by their particular needs and service experiences. Listening to these seniors' struggles and fears may bring up fears for the reader about his or her own future, but the experience should also encourage us to enhance empathy and sensitivity in the care and services we provide.

The first seniors considered in this chapter are living in their own homes, but are willing to talk about the possibility of one day using long-term care services. Next, seniors are considered who continue living in their homes, but now engage a home care worker to assist them. The level and frequency of home care varies from minimal services provided one day a week to more extensive assistance provided every day; all of these seniors have definite preferences about the services they receive. The voices of seniors who have lost their homes and associated independence and are now adjusting to congregate living, either in assisted-living facilities or in nursing homes, are heard subsequently. We hear both seniors at their early moments of loss and listen also to those who have lived in nursing homes for many years. The move to an institution affects family members and loved ones; they may have worried about their parents' safety and feel relief at their move to a more protected environment, yet also feel their parents' losses. Their voices are considered as well.

Hundreds of articles and reports were reviewed for this chapter, but only studies that recorded the actual voices of seniors or their family members are included. These research studies include qualitative interviews that capture concerns and anxieties without the interference of research vocabulary. Rating scales, completed by seniors, depicting ranges of satisfaction or preference are also included. A few studies look at diaries or journals kept by seniors while they used long-term care services. These words are noted in this chapter also.

The narrative that follows provides a context and understanding of the various challenges and perspectives of adults as they age.

Living at Home

Before listening to seniors who actually use long-term care services, we consider the voices of future long-term care consumers. The expectations of middle-aged adults provide insight about support that can be offered in the near future. A greater number of adults are reaching old age with additional financial resources, in better health, and with more education than in any previous generation. Future long-term care users (tomorrow's seniors) have more access to the internet, and surveys show they are comparison shopping and spending more on enhancing their health. These trends can only be expected to continue.[2]

Nearly all surveys reveal that the vast majority of Americans prefer to remain in their homes as they age. Furthermore, many middle-aged adults have modified their homes in the hopes of living there longer or indefinitely. Simple modifications include installing nightlights and putting non-skid strips in bathtubs or showers. Examples of major modifications are installing light switches and handrails in stairwells and making structural changes to facilitate living on the ground floor. Nearly half of these modifications were completed by the homeowners themselves, and 75% of these homeowners believe the modifications will allow them to live in their homes at least another 10 years.[3] These future seniors' expectations are well founded, as studies demonstrate that the most important features that support maintaining independence are a bathroom and bedroom on the main floor of the home, non-slip floors, and covered parking. Neighborhoods, too, are important considerations for seniors living independently. They need to be relatively safe, with health care services located nearby.[4]

Seniors living in their own homes find it difficult admitting that for a variety of reasons they may not be able to remain in their homes. Of seniors admitting this, most have no place in mind for future living. They usually state that they would first modify their homes and try to arrange for services there if faced with physical or cognitive limitations.[5] Of course these adults realize they may need home care assistance in the future. A national survey of adults 55 and older revealed that at least half have already needed home care assistance of some kind. Furthermore, if these adults needed such care today, they could not afford even two hours per day for six months (given the current price of home care services). Merely for financial reasons, the first preference for home assistance is family members. However, forty percent preferred paid help who were not family members, with half wanting to find their own help, and half preferring to pay home care agencies to find and provide their assistants.

Almost a quarter of U.S. households today rely on relatives or friends to provide unpaid home care assistance. About half of these caregivers provide eight hours or less of care per week and about 40% of the seniors receiving such care also have services from a paid assistant, nurse, or housekeeper. Most of these family caregivers do not live with the seniors they care for but live within an hour of driving time and the services requested most from caregiving family members are financial help and transportation. The most popular direct care areas with which family members would like help are in finding easy activities to do with the senior, talking with doctors or other health professionals, finding time for themselves and other family members, and managing emotional stress. Most family members say they initially experience little physical strain, emotional stress, or financial hardship when caregiving, but as the level of care increases, caregiving family members report more and more strain. If family caregivers decide to get help, they most frequently turn to the internet to learn about what treatments and services are available. The second-most popular source of help is their doctor or other health care provider.[6]

Despite not planning on immediate use of home care services, seniors generally agree on certain crucial features of home care services. It is extremely important to most adults that their assistants are honest. Other features of utmost importance to seniors are feeling safe and comfortable with paid assistants, trusting them to come when scheduled, and knowing that they are well trained.[7]

As people age, the probability that they will become disabled increases. Currently, about 40% of people over age 65 have at least some functional limitations which interfere with their daily activities. Surveys of adults with disabilities who live in their own homes provide clues to services seniors need. The number one fear of people with disabilities is loss of independence. Although they have already lost some independence, disabled seniors fiercely want to protect the independence they still have. This often means that they need to have control over how help is provided. As Judith E. Heumann, Co-Founder of World Institute on Disability, states, "Independent living is not doing things by yourself; it is being in control of how things are done."[8]

A national survey of disabled adults revealed many unmet needs that long-term care organizations could address. Some of the things disabled seniors wanted to do but couldn't included paying bills, getting things off of high shelves, tying shoes, getting out of bed, and getting back and forth to the store. Survey respondents stated that they often just did not do these things until a relative or dear friend visited, but they hated their dependence on the unreliable schedules of these loved ones.[9]

Disabled seniors experience losses that affect their quality of life. These areas may not ever be serviced, but reflection on them can provide insight on how better to serve seniors in the future. When asked what they missed most about their pre-disability lives, seniors mentioned simple things such as playing the violin, going fishing, or just going to the park with grandchildren.

These comments reflect the challenges and concerns of people living in the community, primarily without long-term care services. While today we see many seniors receiving supportive services in the home from unpaid family members, population statistics reveal that future generations will not have the level of access to this help that past generations have enjoyed. Services such as home maintenance and the demand for personal services will significantly increase. Fortunately, as the number of seniors grows, their collective power will increase. Voting is the most obvious form this increased power will take, but other powers will also become evident. We can expect to see more legislative proposals which reflect the needs and values of seniors and which may develop into expanded benefits and services.[10]

Home Care Services

Individuals living in their homes who need assistance for maintaining their independence are the primary voices home care organizations hear. The voices of these seniors vary, as some have just started using home care services, some use a homemaker weekly to help with housekeeping or bathing, and others have daily home care attendants to help with the most basic activities of living. Additionally, more and more seniors need home care services only temporarily until they regain their strength and functioning following surgery or an illness. These voices reflect the process of discovering and dealing with failing physical strength and striving to maintain treasured independence at home.

Theodore Roszak suggests that seniors go through a rite of passage as they begin to need services. It is usually initiated by a medical crisis which involves the threat of death. During the crisis and immediately afterward, the senior is excused from all the normal routines of work and family responsibilities. However, during this time he or she loses much dignity, and as he or she becomes healthier, the agonizing reality of lost independence dawns.[11] Generally home care users identify four common concerns—personality and characteristics of home care staff, information and involvement allowed of the senior, specific services and programs provided, and outcomes or results of home care services.

Staff Characteristics

For seniors receiving home care services, the individuals who make home visits—their personalities, their working styles, and their relationships with clients—are the most important concern. The interpersonal and professional skills of these home visit staff profoundly affect how clients evaluate and react to their services. It is not surprising then that staff members (usually nurses and nursing assistants or homemakers) are rigorously critiqued in surveys and interviews.

Seniors expect a home care nurse to perform duties professionally and skillfully, and they expect nursing assistants and homemakers to exhibit strong interpersonal skills. Each staff person, whether a nurse, a therapist, or a homemaker is expected to be caring and listen to them, the client. One focus group discussing home care staff found that the seniors didn't even mention job performance but focused entirely on the interpersonal dynamics of their relationships. The most common complaint was lack of sensitivity on the part of workers.

In one survey of nearly 700 home care clients, excellent staff persons are described as unhurried, clean, on time, and as providing their clients with a sense of self-confidence. One senior stated that her nurse was never too busy to spend time patiently helping her learn how to care for herself. "Very important" characteristics of home care staff are "being thorough and efficient," "taking directions well," "communicating well," "being sensitive," and "being reliable."

Reliable means showing up when scheduled (not being a "no show") and being there for the long run. In a focus group study, one family member said, "Even though our worker was almost always late, we didn't complain—they might send a different one, and I didn't like strangers in my house." One exceptionally reliable homemaker was mentioned as she arranged training for other workers about the senior's individual preferences and style before going on her vacation. Some seniors acknowledged their dependence on their workers and stated this as a reason reliability is so important to them. As one senior said, "If something doesn't get done, it never will; so I need to really depend on [name] to get everything done on her weekly visit."[12]

One study evaluating just homemakers and personal care assistants found that seniors identified ideal characteristics as cheerfulness and trustworthiness. One senior said she preferred "just adequate" care provided by a worker with whom she enjoyed a pleasant relationship to excellent care provided by an unpleasant worker. Professional caregiving style was important too. One particular style was not the issue, but consistency and doing things the client's way were vital concerns. As one client said in a focus group:

> You feel so attached to your nurse. . . .You feel comfortable and confident, then, one day, they send someone else. This nurse puts the equipment in a different place. She took my dad into the bedroom instead of the kitchen. You think, oh no, she's not doing that right, but you know there's nothing you can say bad about the care.[13]

A single, generally preferred working style for homemakers and assistants is impossible to establish as individual seniors have very different preferences in this area. For example, some wanted their worker to "require little direction" while others wanted her to "be willing to take directions." One senior reported she had called her agency requiring another homemaker because the first wasn't willing to take directions. She was much happier with her new worker, who began every visit by asking, "What do you want done most today?" Another senior, however, stated she wanted to leave the directions to the worker and admitted she had grown very passive in her current state of poor health and physical functioning. No one particular work style is preferred, but there must be the flexibility in meeting the seniors' preferred styles of assistance and care.[14]

Several interviewers have found that seniors seemed to value "extras." Extra jobs or tasks the worker did for the senior were often mentioned with clear pride and delight. Examples include assistants picking up groceries on their own time, bringing flowers or vegetables from their gardens, or baking birthday cakes for seniors. One senior reported that once each year her homemaker gathered up several of "us old ladies" and took them shopping. They started with lunch in a cafeteria at the mall, then shopped, and ended the day at an ice cream parlor. All the ladies in her building were envious of her great home care assistant. Other clients described social activities they shared, usually during work time, such as having lunch together, looking at family photos, or dictating and writing letters. In one survey, nearly one-fourth of seniors stated that their worker often stayed extra time and worked longer than paid hours, and nearly 20% reported doing things with their workers outside of work.[15] It may be that seniors value these extras in and of themselves, or it may be that they value the relationships with their assistants that are demonstrated by these activities.

Chatting or socializing during the home visit isn't consistently expected and seems to be contingent on the amount of time workers are scheduled each week. One client who received just one hour of service commented that her worker was too busy during this hour to talk or do much beyond what was absolutely necessary. On the other hand, seniors with live-in workers often mentioned how much they revealed to their workers and the wonderful times they had chatting. Although many of these activities seem like friendship, the reciprocity of friendship was not expected. In one focus group, seniors were asked if having a good relationship entitled their workers to spend time socializing. One senior firmly disagreed: "they should listen and talk while doing things with a purpose."[16]

The "human element" was often emphasized by seniors and described as a compatible relationship. In trying to determine the kinds of relationships seniors expect to have with their assistants, senior clients were asked, "How do you regard the worker—as a friend, a part of your family, as a worker, or what?" Almost two-thirds of clients used informal terms such as "friend" or "like family." Others spoke of the companionship they have found with their workers describing them as their windows to the world. Workers were often the only people seniors saw during the day or, sometimes, during the week. Many confessed they had told their workers private matters that they hadn't even told their children. Nearly three-fourths of the seniors discussed personal problems with their workers. For these seniors, the least important characteristics were punctuality and doing extras or work outside the job description.[17]

Information and Involvement

Not being informed about necessary care and availability of agency services was the most frequent problem experienced by home care clients and their family members. It also was identified as the second-most important driver of dissatisfaction among home care consumers. Many seniors remembered coming home from the hospital confused and afraid. They had many questions they had forgotten to ask and were worried not only about their healing procedures, but also about doing everyday activities. Several family members remembered wondering when the first home visits would occur and worrying what the nurses would be like. Some seniors realized that nurses may have given them information at the hospital, but in their nervousness about going home, they just couldn't recall. Most seniors insisted that hospital health care directions and information were inadequate. Some reported that their agencies had on-call nurses available by telephone to respond to such questions, and all the seniors in the discussion group thought that sounded like a wonderful service.

In addition to being informed, family members stressed how important it was for seniors to be involved in their own care and in monitoring their own progress. Either the senior or a family member must be capable of doing all necessary medical techniques at home because "it was only you for most of the day and night." In one focus group, the wife of an elderly home care client stressed to the group how important it was to practice such techniques while the nurse was there. She informed the other seniors of her belief that the nurse should allow them to practice over and over. "If the nurse is in a hurry. . .you feel bad to ask her again . . .but if you don't, you'll suffer later."[18]

The amount of control clients have over their attendants is another area of involvement. The younger disabled populations typically have more control over their home care attendants' scheduling and procedural styles; they also have the responsibility of hiring, firing, and training their home care attendants. However, surveys reveal that the majority of seniors (78%) do not want this type of control. Seniors state that they were willing to *accept* more control if necessary, but would not pursue it. Specific aspects of control seniors are most willing to assume responsibility for are scheduling and supervising. Areas seniors are not so willing to control are hiring and firing workers, although nearly 30% are willing to hire and 24% are willing to fire their workers. [19]

Home care services mediated by case managers, who authorize the services and develop care plans specifying how, when, and by whom care will be provided (all within specific budgets) have been examined for client satisfaction. In one study, about a quarter of the seniors stated they could take more responsibility for the supervision and direction of their own care, and about a third could cope with less case manager involvement.[20] Interestingly, very few seniors had any experience in hiring domestic help, and they requested training in this area if the care manager program was to be eliminated or downsized. While it may seem that clients do not want more control, clients with the most choice and control do report the highest levels of satisfaction. This suggests that satisfaction is associated with greater involvement in all aspects of managing an attendant.

Another home care study found that providing multiple channels of information as a means of empowering clients was a major factor in distinguishing excellent from merely satisfactory home care.[21] Both client and family member involvement in care decisions and staff understanding of care goals were hallmarks of the home care agencies rated as "excellent." Staff members were reported as providing clear explanations of care, procedures, and medications, and permitting time for and encouraging questions. Part of the involvement and education of the client involved orientation to home care.[22] Primarily, this means that the senior knows whom to call with questions and whom to contact for immediate attention. These actions seemed to empower the senior and his or her family members in dealing with excellent home care agencies.

Preferred Services

Seniors using home care services identify two specific services as frequently needed: housekeeping services and on-call nursing to answer questions between home visits. Housekeeping services are the most common unmet need clients mention when discussing their home care. Several seniors were managing fine during the interviews, but stated that when they first arrived home from the hospital, housekeeping duties were really needed. In other surveys, seniors described unmet housekeeping needs as a constant strain because home care assistants did not include them in their care plans (it is not a reimbursed service in many states). Other seniors stated they did not know what they would do without the help of family members doing household chores.

Lack of on-call professionals to contact with health questions was a frequent complaint among seniors and their family members. Agencies that provided this service were highly praised, and seniors felt much more confident in their ability to function at home just knowing that professionals were only a phone call away. In focus groups, when an agency was mentioned that provided this service, all seniors asked for the name and number of this agency.[23]

Residential Living / Assisted-Living Facilities

Some seniors desire a residential environment that combines health care and support services so that as they grow frail or their disabilities increase, they are able to maintain a higher level of independence and dignity than is often possible in traditional nursing homes. Assisted-living facilities, independent-living facilities, and other supported residential facilities are the initial structures meeting this desire. Today, these types of facilities comprise one of the fastest-growing segments of the long-term care industry. However, with their minimal regulations, these facilities vary greatly in their structures, services, and clients. Research, too, is scant, in part because national or even regional identification of facilities is difficult, and facilities in one state may be labeled as independent-living, while in another state they are called assisted-living or group homes. Generally, however, over half of the seniors living in these facilities are in their late eighties and need assistance with one or more major activity of daily living (bathing, dressing, transferring, toileting, and eating). Some need assistance with only one of these activities, while others need help with two or three, and a small percent need help with more than three. Other needs with which some seniors need help include ambulating, incontinence care, and needs that emerge at various stages of dementia.[24]

When seniors on a waiting list for either an independent-living facility or continuing care retirement community were asked why they were willing to move, the majority reported a desire to have health care available if needed. Other important reasons seniors gave for moving included no longer having household maintenance chores and assuring they did not become a burden on their families.[25] Similar reasons for moving were found in another study of seniors living in a continuing care retirement community. About 40% cited preferences for their place of death as playing a role in their decision to move. They wanted care available if necessary for a terminal illness, they did not want to be a burden to their families, and they did not want to die alone.[26]

Surveys regarding the importance of various features and services reveal a variance in opinions between new consumers and those who had lived in a facility for at least one year. For new consumers, personal security and the availability of medical care are the most important considerations. Other features rated as very important are meals, nursing staff, location near relatives, and reputation for providing quality care. [27, 28, 29] For family members who had recently selected congregate care facilities for their relatives, the most critical consideration in their final selection was the attitude of the staff. The next most important features were location close to them and excellent nursing care.[30]

Seniors living in assisted-living or other independent-living type facilities consistently report high overall satisfaction. Only a few studies identity specific areas of satisfaction and dissatisfaction. Actually, satisfaction with assisted-living or other independent residential facilities is found to be influenced more by the personal characteristics of seniors than by any facility feature or service. Seniors with few disabilities and happy dispositions who felt they controlled the decision to relocate to the facility are most highly satisfied with their residential facility, regardless of its size, organizational structure, or other amenities and services.[31] It appears that about half of seniors moving into assisted-living facilities feel they have complete control over facility selection, while about 25% feel they have little or no control.[32]

A few specific aspects of care or services have been identified when seniors are asked for suggestions to improve their facility or other ingenious questions. Food and meal-time features, as well as staff characteristics, are mentioned by seniors in all studies. Seniors more frequently voice their complaints about a variety of aspects of these services, while a few seniors provide suggestions for improvements. Recreational services were an area about which seniors are not particularly pleased but they found it difficult to suggest specific improvements.

Staff Characteristics

Seniors have both positive and negative things to say about their nursing assistants. Most seniors rate their assistants high in treating them with dignity, and about half believe their assistants take time to listen to them. However, all studies found that the majority of seniors believe there are not enough assistants to care for all the seniors for whom they are given responsibility. Several seniors noted that assistants seem to try hard, but that they often experience very long waits for getting help.

About 50% of seniors mention that they do not think assistants have much training or that they are poorly supervised. Sometimes seniors complained regarding how assistants provided care and wondered who taught the assistants or whom to speak to about changing the way assistance was provided. These concerns, however, often were blamed on the low number of assistants in a facility. Nearly three-fourths of seniors believe their facilities had trouble retaining good staff. Seniors identified characteristics of good assistants as being genuinely concerned, kind, respectful, and consistently attentive. Some seniors thought it was important for nursing assistants to have pleasant dispositions, and these seniors did not want staff bringing their problems to work.

As previously mentioned, most seniors prefer to stay in their independent care facilities, and many greatly feared nursing homes. This fear has the potential to intimidate seniors into staying in "independent" facilities which provide inadequate or unsafe care. One study of seniors living in assisted-living facilities showed the seniors video scenarios of different types of staff abuse and asked them to (a) identify the type of abuse and (b) identify what they would do if they experienced this type of abuse. Most seniors could identify physical, fiduciary, and medication-assistance abuse, but most did not identify verbal abuse, neglect, or environmental hazards. Furthermore, half of the seniors did not know what they would do if they experienced these types of abuse. Of those seniors who came up with responses, half said they would call on family members.[33]

Preferred Services

The quality of food and of meal-time experiences are common complaints. It is clear that it is impossible to please all palates. In the same facility, some seniors complained food was too spicy, while others complained it was too bland. Only a quarter of seniors in assisted-living facilities rated the food as always tasty. Many seniors complained that no appealing alternatives were offered if they didn't like the food served at a particular meal. In one survey a daughter stated that an alternative sandwich took over an hour to prepare but was still frozen in the middle. Many facilities seem to have a fairly structured dinner service with table companions and places assigned. One senior stated that he felt he was destined to eat with the same persons for the remainder of his life.[34]

Recreational activities and services vary, both by the type of seniors living in a facility and by the staff in charge of this program. A survey of assisted-living facilities found that about half of seniors participate in most of the planned activities and about that many enjoy them most of the time. The other seniors participate in a few activities but generally are not interested in the planned events. Again, about half of the seniors in assisted-living facilities are not consulted regarding preferred activities. The most frequently requested recreational activity in all assisted-living surveys was transportation on individual trips within the community. Some seniors want to shop in specific stores, others want to visit community friends, and some want to attend specific events. Most seniors either did not want to bother family members or did not have close relatives to ask for transportation help. Most seniors in assisted-living facilities did participate in group outings outside their facilities and enjoyed getting out into the community. However, many seniors wanted the opportunity to continue seeing old friends or participating in community events just as they did prior to moving. However, they didn't want to go places with a "crowd of old people." [35]

Outcomes

Most seniors in assisted-living facilities hope their facilities will be their last home on earth and that they will not be moved to nursing homes. As previously stated, many seniors select their supported residential facilities partly to prevent dying alone and to avoid burdening family. Unfortunately, if a senior does not die there, the most likely outcome is transfer to a nursing home, usually because the seniors needs more care than the facility can provide. Despite these concerns, the majority of seniors living in these facilities do not know the criteria for discharge or at what point in their disabilities and care needs the residential facility would tell them they must leave.[36]

Nursing Homes

Nursing homes are the original residential institutions for seniors who can no longer live independently in the community. They have been labeled as sterile and rigid facilities, and seniors are known to dread the prospect of living in one. Fortunately, these facilities have changed quite a bit from the facilities of the '70s and '80s; however, many improvements can still be made. Generally, nursing homes provide more encompassing care for people with severe medical needs and disabilities, and seniors who live in these facilities have a higher degree of functional, health, and cognitive impairments. Surprisingly, nursing homes also provide more social and recreational services than other types of facilities.[37] On the negative side, nursing homes provide significantly less privacy, with few private rooms or baths. The acceptance of seniors with behavioral problems as residents also provides less comfort for many seniors who are also living in the facilities. Listening to the voices of seniors living in these facilities provides administrators much more insight than surveys of these facilities' policies or survey results.

Staff Characteristics

Just as with other services, caring, responsive staff are unequivocally the most important component of nursing home care. In the seminal study conducted by the *National Citizens' Coalition for Nursing-Home Reform*, not only was good staff the top priority of seniors throughout the United States, but also staff characteristics and styles of providing care were mentioned more than any other areas—617 times in the 135 discussion groups.[38] Several studies now empirically demonstrate that the seniors' evaluations of staff behaviors are significantly related to an individual nursing home's survey results.[39]

Along with some of the same personal characteristics of staff discussed previously, the words "adequate numbers" and "more staff" were frequently heard. Having sufficient staff, positive staff attitudes, and good relationships with staff were the issues seniors raised most often. Seniors emphasized the importance of having qualified, well-trained, and well-supervised staff.

When seniors were asked what could be done to improve the quality of staff, responses clustered into two areas: attitudes and performance. For performance seniors frequently identified the need for staff to receive training to perform specific care tasks ranging from personal care (denture care, dressing assistance) to basic nursing skills (bowel and bladder training, walking assistance). Seniors also focused on the need for more supervision and orientation and the importance of finding and hiring qualified staff. Many seniors saw increased pay as one way to achieve this. In the area of attitudes, seniors felt that staff should learn to communicate better with clients. Communication and its role in overcoming social isolation came up in several later studies as significant needs. Treating seniors with respect, listening to them, and responding to requests without complaints were important considerations. Not surprisingly, seniors also identified a pleasant disposition as important in caregivers. Many seniors stated they wanted the assistants to smile at least once in awhile.[40]

Seniors in several studies report missing communication "from the heart." The absence of "someone to talk with from the staff" was reported as a significant problem both in nursing homes with high quality ratings and in those with poor ratings. One study used a variety of scenarios in which seniors indirectly voiced their anger, worry, or depression to the nurses. Seniors then stated how they thought their nurses would react. No matter how good the home, a large proportion of seniors felt nurses would not encourage communication about depression or loss. In better-rated homes, more seniors felt their nurses would respond to worries or angry feelings and encourage the seniors to talk about their feelings. Overall, however, a large percentage of seniors felt their nurses would not encourage this level of communication.[41]

Some studies found feelings of social isolation and loneliness correlated with seniors' feeling they were burdening nursing staff. In many nursing homes, seniors could not identify anyone they were close to among the staff. A study in Denmark found that nursing home seniors who preferred to return to their community homes reported significantly more social isolation than those who preferred to stay in the nursing home.[42] Staff empathy and responsiveness could alleviate much of the social isolation seniors felt. Seniors identified these qualities by expressing their beliefs that staff gave them personal attention, worked with *their* needs at heart, and could be trusted to keep confidences. Studies of American nursing homes found that in homes where residents rated staff as highly nurturing there were fewer official complaints and survey deficiencies.[43]

Senior-staff interactions at all levels create a climate or atmosphere that can be warm and accepting or lonely and socially isolating. Staff behavior, as well as words, can unconsciously create an overall atmosphere that influences how seniors feel about themselves, how they behave, and how they relate to others. Berdes points out that no matter how good nursing homes are, they still are by their nature an unintentional opportunity for dehumanizing and isolating seniors.[44] Dehumanization is not something staff members intentionally do to seniors, but rather the cumulative effect of communication, behavior, and organizational norms. This is often labeled the social atmosphere or climate of a facility and it can be supportive and comforting or isolating and cruel.

Components of social climate measured in nursing homes are cohesion and conflict among seniors and staff, the degree of independence seniors feel, and the level of comfort and control seniors feel. The cohesion dimension includes feelings of helpfulness from staff towards seniors, the degree of supportiveness of seniors with one other, and the extent to which seniors are critical and express anger. The independence dimension includes how self-sufficient seniors are encouraged to be and how openly they are encouraged to express themselves. Homes to which seniors gave poor social climate ratings were also rated significantly lower by outside evaluators than those described as having good social climates. The researchers felt that the social climate of an institution can promote health or destroy initiative and independence. Incidentally, this was found true not only for seniors, but also for the staff; this finding will be elaborated on in the next chapter.[45]

Information and Involvement

A sense of control over who one is and what one does is perhaps the most fundamental feature of a meaningful life. In order to achieve this control, individuals need information about the choices available to them and the possible consequences of each. A life with the option of making uninformed choices is little better than a passive, dehumanizing existence.

Information and involvement should be part of the decision to enter a residential care home. Seniors need to have visited the home prior to admission, have exhausted all available options, and have determined that the move to a particular home is their choice. This involvement and decision making process is important to seniors not only at the initial admission to a home, but also has been found to significantly impact "nursing home adjustment" years later. One study found that nursing home residents who believed their move to a nursing home was voluntary were better adjusted than those who felt they had no control over their move to the home.[46] Another study of seniors living in nursing homes who were asked if they preferred to return home or stay, found that the attitude seniors had on admission strongly predicted their preference up to ten years later. In other words, those who had not wanted to go into a nursing home in the first place showed distinct signs of not adjusting and preferring to move out.[47]

Once in a nursing home, seniors want to be involved in many matters impacting daily life. The most popular area of interest is food and meals. Other areas where involvement is desired are activities of daily living such as personal bathing preferences and being able to use a washing machine and dryer to wash their own clothes. Keeping pets and plants in their rooms or nursing home lobbies was an area over which seniors had lost control and dearly missed. The National Coalition study found that over half of seniors want to make choices about their food. They also want to choose when to get up and to go to bed and have assistance to come and go as they please. Other significant areas of daily life in which seniors want some choice include which activities to participate in, choice of roommates, and time of bath.[48]

Seniors provide several suggestions to make staff more responsive to residents' choices. The first set of suggestions involved staff allowing group participation in decisions, making changes in staff attitudes, and supporting seniors in being more assertive. Specific suggestions include disciplining staff, letting the seniors evaluate staff, providing more supervision and administrative checks, and making administration more responsive to seniors' choices. Additional suggestions included involving seniors in board meetings, involving family, taking seniors' complaints more seriously, allowing seniors to sit where they would like to in the dining room, having staff support seniors in choices, acting on senior council suggestions, making staff accountable to senior councils, and having staff ask seniors questions directly as well as surveying seniors. Seniors also mentioned wanting to have more night staff to help dress for bed, more help with personal tasks, as well as to have their own phones and their own visitors.[49]

Preferred Services

Services and program preferences are fairly consistent throughout studies of nursing home seniors and their family members. Some of the recommended services are similar to those recommended in other long-term care programs. Family involvement, food service changes, and additional recreational services seem to be consistent themes.

Interviews with family members of nursing home seniors reveal that they feel they play an integral and critical part in improving seniors' quality of life and care. In fact, most families are convinced that a senior without involved relatives has a lower quality of life and care.[50] Most family members focus primarily on meeting the social and emotional needs of their relative; however, a few play major roles in overall advocacy and monitoring. Family members are often involved with providing for their relatives' social and emotional needs, communicating regularly with staff and administration, and performing surprise visits to monitor care. Many are engaged in monitoring the care of other seniors without family advocates, encouraging the use of volunteers to meet needs, ensuring that personal care plans are followed, seeing to it that seniors exercise, alerting staff to physical changes and needs, and helping feed seniors at meals.

The major concerns family members identify are poor communication among staff, seniors, and family members; lack of trust regarding care; failure of staff to maintain seniors' dignity; and staff discouraging or preventing family from maintaining connectedness. The need for dignity was often mentioned. One daughter noted that staff had unconscious infantilizing habits of addressing seniors with unearned terms of endearment: "honey," "love," "sweetie," and "dear." She found these terms patronizing and "wounding to the spirit."[51]

One suggestion from family members is that administrators develop policies and programs to orient, support, and develop families as an important resource in collaboratively providing technical and preservative care.[52] One researcher who read multiple nursing home seniors' diaries recommends that no one at a home be without outside contacts.[53] If no family member is close, a paid advocate should be appointed on admission. The family member or advocate will agree to visit a certain number of times per month, take the senior out of the home several times per year, and participate in care planning and the delivery of other personal services.

Food ranked third among the quality factors brought up in the first round of discussion groups, and again, all groups mentioned food issues.[54] In response to the question, "What would make food service good in a nursing home?" seniors ranked variety first, hot food second, and choices including a menu third. Specific food preferences, such as fresh fruits and vegetables and seasonings, were common among the groups. Others requested reasonably sized portions, attractively served meals, and provisions for special dietary needs.

The seniors seemed well aware of the value of dieticians and the need for professional planning and supervision of food preparation. Many indicated they were aware of good nutritional practices and wanted them followed. Seniors were asked what it would take to make good food happen. While one senior said that it would take a miracle, most thought choice should be the first priority followed by variety, seasonings, timely service, faster preparation, better quality supervision, and cooperation among all. A fourth area of discussion was to revise the food system creatively for better organization of service. Other creative ideas offered included fishing, raising chickens and other animals to eat, and providing gardens or window boxes in which to grow fresh vegetables.

From the point of view of many seniors, if food service is to be improved in nursing homes, seniors must have input in the planning and implementation of food service programs. Respondents often complained that foods were not warm enough and that the menus lacked variety. They felt that staff and administration could improve things in these areas. One senior stated, "The menu reads well, but the preparation is atrocious, and complaints go unheeded."[55]

Studies of both seniors and family members find that they want expanded activity options. The most popular options were social activities, games, and activities outside the home. Outside activities included shopping trips, field trips, outings for scenic and cultural events, and eating in restaurants.

Arts and crafts and "activities that use your mind" were suggested. Arts and crafts noted included sewing, ceramics, and other table work. Mind activities included keeping up with current events and history, access to books, and reading discussions. However, these were not quite as popular as the aforementioned activities. One daughter said, "My mother is still a bright and mentally alert person and needs more challenges than bingo and basket weaving."[56] Some family members want physical activity on a regular schedule and more one-to-one encouragement of their relative. "It would be nice if staff would come around to encourage and maybe even assist in the activity room."[57]

In several surveys, seniors stated that choice was an important component of the activities program. They wanted choices regarding what to attend, when, and their degree of participation. Many seniors said they would like activities to be scheduled on evenings and weekends. One senior stated, "I would like to see a better activity curriculum. It seems that after 8:00 P.M. they roll up the sidewalks, so to speak." [58] Seniors identified contributing factors to a successful activity program as a dynamic activities director, adequate staff, more volunteers, and cooperation among departments. Also stressed was participation of the community at large. This included suggestions for transportation or volunteer transporters. Several seniors wanted to visit frail friends outside the facility and wanted individual transportation arranged.

As important as recreation services are, they should be put in perspective. In one national study, they were rated fourth in importance, after staff, environment, and food. In another study, the highest-rated nursing home had all the best qualities of theses attributes; however, the second best-rated home had everything else, but few recreational activities, while lower-rated homes had more recreational services, but less congenial staff.

Conclusion

Clearly zest for life and desire for independence do not fade as seniors start to use long-term care services. A struggle to maintain some control is witnessed in every setting—from seniors remodeling and living alone in their own homes, to seniors dependent on home care assistants to help them out of bed, to seniors living in facilities who want to control when they get up and what they eat. Disabilities force seniors to give up much, but control over their own care is not given up lightly. The most consistent worry among seniors receiving any type of long-term care is who will provide care for them. Seniors want kind, considerate, and caring staff who will take the time to treat them as individuals, not as another bed to make. They also consistently voice concern about the amount of work expected of assistants and the inadequate staff ratios.

These are the voices of seniors who are served or will be served in long-term care. The individual staff member, especially assistants or nurses' aides, is the senior's closest most constant companion. In the next chapter we listen to them as they work in each of the settings identified here and as they perceive the seniors they care for and the professionals to whom they report.

 C3 80

Discussion Questions

1. The majority of boomers and aging adults want to stay in their own homes as they age. What are some activities in which they could engage in order to achieve this goal?

2. Many middle aged individuals, as well as seniors, have modified their homes to permit themselves to live in them as they become disabled. How will this trend impact future long-term care organizations? What additional services may be needed to serve future generations of seniors?

3. Home care services are expensive on a long term basis, with the majority of seniors being able to afford only 2 days a week for 6 months. Provide suggestions to make this service more affordable to seniors.

4. Compatibility between frontline workers and seniors is very important in home care services. However, there is not one style of worker that works best for all seniors. Each senior has his or her own preference. What then, as an administrator hiring frontline workers, would you look for in assistants?

5. Compare general characteristics of seniors using home care agencies with seniors using supported residential facilities, other than nursing homes. What services and resources would be similar for these long-term care organizations? What services and resources would differ between these organizations?

6. List the reasons seniors give for moving into a supported residential facility and the features seniors consider very important once they have lived in a residential facility. How can seniors (and their family members) act as savvy consumers to investigate these significant features before they move into a facility? Provide suggestions for consumer reports in these areas. How would information be obtained? Where would it be reported?

7. One study of seniors living is assisted-living facilities revealed that most seniors could not identify verbal abuse, neglect, or environmental hazards. Furthermore, half of the seniors did not know what they would do if they experienced these types of abuse. One of the worries mentioned with this study is that seniors may be living in fear of being sent to a nursing home and thus refuse to complain. Provide a variety of strategies that a caring administrator could use to avoid or overcome this potential problem.

8. Identify volunteer opportunities available in home care services, assisted-living facilities, and nursing homes. Identify the skills and resources needed for these volunteer positions. Create job descriptions for these positions. Can any of these positions overlap? What would be some incentives and some disincentives for an administrator regarding overlapping volunteers into more than one long-term care setting?

9. Several studies found that nursing home residents missed communicating their real feelings with staff. In fact, a large proportion of seniors feel nursing staff would not encourage communication about their depression or loss, which contributes to feelings of isolation and loneliness. How can an administrator encourage heart-felt communication in order to help seniors overcome the feelings of isolation they experience?

10. Nursing home residents made several suggestions to make staff more responsive to them. Some of these suggestions included letting the residents evaluate staff, involving residents in board meetings, and taking residents' complaints more seriously. Consider these suggestions and then respond to how they could be implemented. Provide other suggestions to help staff be more responsive to seniors.

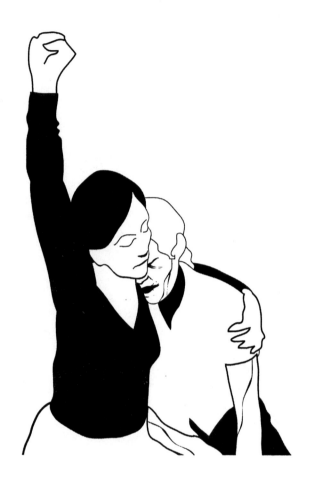

"I help my family triumph over personal hardships
and give comfort to suffering seniors."

CHAPTER 3

VOICES OF FRONTLINE STAFF

"I was so pumped up when I was hired. It was totally different when I got on the floor. I love what I do but I get so discouraged. If you can't get respect, go for the money... A bunch of us will go talk to administration. They say they'll look into it—and that's the last you hear about your issue." [1]

Frontline staff members are defined as the primary workers in any long-term care organization, whether home care, nursing home or assisted-living facility. This chapter considers their voices and perspectives. Whether they are called nursing assistants, home care assistants, or direct care workers, they provide the care and daily services seniors depend on. A smile, an extra moment, or other recognition from a daily caregiver can make all the difference in a lonely senior's day. In contrast, experiencing a gruff remark, hurried manner, or a distracted facial expression can leave a senior discouraged and disheartened.

Beyond these staff members' demeanors, the services they provide are essential. They ensure that seniors enjoy clean environments, whether in nursing home rooms or in their own homes. They provide nutritional nourishment by shopping, preparing meals, or actually feeding ailing seniors. Most important, frontline staff render personal hygiene and comfort services including bathing, making beds and, at times, assisting with toileting. Last, assistants are often seniors' sole channels to the outside world, bringing information about events and news to homebound or institutionalized seniors who might otherwise not be aware of such things.

Nationwide, there are at least 2 million frontline staff who provide care to those living in their homes, assisted-living facilities, group homes, and nursing homes.[2] Nearly 90 percent of these caregivers are women with low incomes and few support systems (e.g., friends or family they can count on).[3] Many are unmarried heads of household with dependent children, 33% are African American and approximately 15% are either Hispanic or other workers of color. Their average age range is 39 years, although they range in age from 20 to 70 years. Wages for these frontline workers are very low, even when compared with other low-wage jobs. Many frontline workers live paycheck to paycheck, holding multiple jobs to make ends meet. (In 2000, nursing assistants in nursing homes earned an average of $8.29 per hourly wage compared to $9.22 for other service workers, and the median income for service workers was $13,287 per year while the median income for home care workers was $12,265 per year.)[4] Furthermore, few of these positions provide health care benefits. In fact, the trend is that these positions are losing health care coverage more quickly than other workers in the U.S.[5]

Training requirements for frontline staff are quite varied. Federal law requires Medicare-funded certified nurse assistants and home health assistants to receive 75 hours of training, and pass a certification exam and skills test. The necessary skills to pass the competency test range from basic communication and documentation skills to knowledge of emergency procedures, transfer techniques, and methods in personal care. Each year these frontline staff must have 12 hours of in-service education, with some states requiring additional hours of training annually. Personal assistants or home care assistants do not have a required federal training standard, but several states require some minimum level of demonstrated competency.

Despite the fact that these assistants provide about 80% of all care within long-term care organizations, their voices and attitudes are difficult to ascertain. Yet these individuals' attitudes, values, and behaviors significantly influence the quality of life for many seniors. Administrators cannot provide support to these essential staff members without hearing and understanding their perspectives. They must first fully understand and appreciate assistants in order to manage them effectively. They are, after all, the backbone as well as the heart and soul of the long-term care industry.

As in the preceding chapter, hundreds of articles and reports related to the work of frontline assistants were reviewed, but only studies that recorded the actual voices of nursing assistants are included here. In some studies researchers interviewed nursing assistants and in others researchers observed their interactions with seniors. Studies in which researchers observed assistants for long periods of time and recorded behaviors as well as conversations are included. In these studies, researchers worked as nursing assistants to more closely observe and come to understand frontline work day-to-day. A few studies placed observers in corners to watch and record assistants' behaviors and words.

Each type of study contributes to building a complete portrait of frontline assistants. The survey methods using either yes or no responses or the Likert scale of ranking a response from 1 to 5 provide the ability statistically to determine the consistency of responses. The qualitative methods of face-to-face interviews and focus groups allow for follow-up questions to obtain clarifications, probing when necessary to get a thorough response to the question. Considering the results of all of these methods provides a fairly complete portrait of frontline staff and their critical roles in long-term care services.

Nursing Home Assistant

Nursing home assistants' work is physically and emotionally demanding. Lifting and transferring people to and from chairs or beds is hard work, and often assistants must also deal with bitter and hostile comments from nursing home residents who are irritable. Some confused nursing home residents actively fight assistants trying to bathe or toilet them. One assistant said of her confused residents, "They curse you, scratch you, and bite you."[6]

In a nursing home, a typical assistant's day starts with waking the residents, getting them up and preparing them for breakfast and medications, usually all within the first hour.[7] Several assistants noted that this morning job was the hardest part of the day. The hour was early for the residents, and they often fought getting up. Many assistants believed that seniors should be able to sleep in, but that they needed to follow the rules of the facility. So assistants would joke with and cajole the grumpiest seniors. Tasks were even more frustrating when supplies, such as diapers, bed linen, or towels were not available or in short supply. This seemed to happen often in some facilities.

The rest of a typical day consisted of feeding, toileting, bathing, and assisting residents to lie down for a nap or to participate in specific activities. Each day, the nursing assistants hoped they did not get assigned too many "feeders" as that tended to really slow work. ("Feeders" are seniors needing someone to assist them with eating or to spoon-feed them.) Assistants performed tasks such as giving showers and bed baths, helping residents with toileting, and making beds; all their work was accomplished under time pressure. For the day shift, the rush was to complete this work before lunch, and for the evening shift, the assistants needed to complete work before bedtime.

The majority of nursing assistants work more than 40 hours a week. Some try to work a specific number of double shifts, others work part-time at second jobs and still others work two full-time jobs. Most work two shifts in nursing homes or in a combination of home care and nursing home jobs. For these double-duty assistants, the first shift often starts near 5:00 A.M. and the second shift or home-visit schedule generally starts around 3:30 P.M. Often assistants leave their homes before dawn and return after dark, hoping to keep their punishing schedules just long enough to get them over some temporary financial hurdles. Some figure exactly how many extra shifts they must work per month. For example, in one study, a new assistant discovered that her full-time take home pay for the month would cover only three weeks' rent. She worked one extra week each month to make ends meet.[8]

Assisted-Living Facility Assistant

Assistants in assisted-living facilities (ALF) do not need the certification that nursing home assistants do; nevertheless, most of them are certified to dispense medications. The morning shift of an ALF assistant starts similarly to that of most nursing home assistants; however, the chores seem to be a blend of home care with nursing home care duties. Observation in one small assisted-living facility provides some insight.[9] During this observation, 14 seniors resided in the facility and two assistants were working there. For the first two hours, one assistant fixed a warm breakfast for everyone and prepared the lunch, putting it in the oven to bake. The other assistant was responsible for seeing that all clients got up for breakfast, were dressed, and got out of their rooms for a while. Some seniors were very independent and did not need help. For those seniors, the assistant tried to watch when they were in the kitchen eating breakfast, so that she could rush in and clean their rooms. About half of the seniors needed a little assistance with dressing, and some of the women asked for final touches on their hair or make-up. The assistant who managed the cooking then prepared the medications and dispensed them to the seniors. Breakfast was on each senior's schedule within about a 2-hour time span.

Bathing or showering the seniors who were on the bath schedule that day took up the next few hours before lunch. Also during this time, the assistants finished cleaning rooms and bathrooms and doing the laundry for the seniors. Some had scheduled appointments with community health professionals during this time, and the assistants made sure to transport the seniors on time. In addition, the assistants noted a problem with one senior's eye and called to schedule an appointment with an ophthalmologist. The pharmacist called, and the assistant faxed a new medication order to him. The morning seemed to fly by for the assistants with such a variety of duties, and soon they began lunch preparations.

Lunch was ready by 11:30. With the seniors helping set the tables, everyone was eating by noon. While the seniors ate, the assistants helped them with cutting food or opening containers. None of the seniors needed actual help with using the utensils. One senior requested something else to eat. The assistant reviewed the leftovers in the refrigerator, and selected something to be warmed up. One assistant then prepared and dispensed the next round of medications. After lunch, one assistant left, and the remaining assistant washed up the dishes, prepared the supper meal and put it in the oven. Many of the seniors took naps in the afternoon, but one or two seniors were always up in the activity / living room. With the kitchen duties done, the assistant prepared an activity and presented it to the seniors, providing support and instructions as needed. This assistant receives a monthly activity magazine at the facility and uses it for arts and crafts ideas. Yet during the afternoon, she also just had conversations with the seniors, helped some of them with writing letters and read mail to those who needed help. The assistant said that everyday she makes sure some music is on and tries to stimulate the seniors into dance movements or to at least talk about social events they used to enjoy.

The evening shift had one assistant for 14 residents. The assistant served the dinner, dispensed medications, and washed dishes. Seniors decided when they wanted to go to their rooms and would let the assistant know. She then either accompanied the senior to help undress or waited about 20 minutes and came into the senior's room to check on him or her. During the evening hours, the assistant gave many of the seniors' individual attention. For some it was a short checkers game and for others it was a conversation, help with letter writing, or just listening to some reminiscing. Any laundry that was not completed in the daytime was finished up in the evening hours. After helping all seniors with their needs, the night shift assistant did what meal preparation she could for the next day. She checked the medication updates and did a variety of paper work that needed completion. If the daytime assistant left a note regarding preparations needed for a craft project, the night assistant organized the materials.

Home Care Assistant

Bob Herbert titled one of his New York Times columns, "The Invisible Women." In this article, he describes home health assistants: "They are the invisible women who fan out across the city each day, mostly traveling by subway, to go into people's homes and do the grunt work of caring for those who are sick or infirm."[10] For every senior in a nursing home or assisted-living facility, two or more equally impaired seniors live in their homes in the community. Home care assistants can be a home health assistant and therefore trained to provide some health care services (under the supervision of a nurse who visits on her own) or can be a home care assistant who provides help with activities of daily living (ADLs) and more general work such as housekeeping, meal preparation, shopping, and bill paying. Often home health care assistants will also do the work of a home care assistant, merging the two positions when necessary.

In following one home health care assistant from her first visit at 7:30 A.M. to her last visit at 5:00 P.M., it was found that her tasks were quite similar to those done in assisted-living facilities and nursing homes.[11] However, in addition to personal care tasks such as bathing, washing hair, and taking vital signs, the home care assistant also performed housekeeping, cooking, and shopping tasks. The assistant showered all attention on each individual senior, thus conversations were more personal and caring than those observed in a nursing home. The job pressure seemed to stem from all the tasks needing completion in the limited time allowed for each home visit. The consequent rush seemed to bother some assistants, especially when they knew the seniors they were caring for had no other visitors for the day.

One researcher who followed a New York City home care assistant described her as a social worker, confidante, nurse, and manager of the home environment.[12] This assistant's day started with the first home visit at 9:00 A.M. to an elderly woman with congestive heart failure who had just gotten home after a week's hospitalization. The assistant fixed breakfast, washed the dishes, bathed her client, took her vital signs, and prepared lunch. A neighbor relieved her after two hours, and she traveled to the second client. There she found no food, so she went grocery shopping, prepared and ate lunch with her client. While eating, she found out her third client was canceled because of an unexpected hospitalization. Therefore, the assistant gathered her current client's laundry and took it to the local laundry room, chatted, and played cards with her senior client as she seemed lonely. Her extra caring was done without recognition or reimbursement. After this visit, she went to her agency to chart and pick up her paycheck at 3:00 P.M.

Daily Functions

The following sections refer to the variety of front line assistants, just described—home care assistants, nursing home assistants and assisted-living assistants. Common functions identified as activities most frontline assistants do every day with multiple seniors include functional care, psychosocial or custodial care, and nourishment tasks; such workers often display efficient work styles and engage in extra initiatives and, sometimes, abusive activities. Several of these activities do overlap, such as functional care and psychosocial care. Other activities, such as "extra initiatives" are performed by the best frontline assistants, while abusive activities are recognized as being committed by only a small percentage of assistants. An efficient work style was recognized as necessary if the frontline worker was to survive in his or her position for long.

The actual tasks nursing assistants perform are important, but just as important as these tasks are how they feel about them. A great deal of personal insight and sensitivity is necessary to accurately recognize feelings towards those with whom one has daily interactions, such as family members, co-workers, or dependent clients. Conflicting values, physical or emotional exhaustion, and co-dependency may all complicate assistants' emotions about their clients. To gain the most accurate understanding of assistants' behaviors towards clients, studies are examined that involved both direct and indirect questions and both recorded and analyzed comments, behaviors, and even facial expressions directed toward clients. The results reveal both the spoken and the unspoken voices of nursing assistants. Shared next are actions, as well as feelings and thoughts behind these functions.

Functional Care

Nursing home assistants, identified as "expert assistants" by their charge nurses, describe functional care best. These assistants were asked to describe the types of care they gave and how they contributed to high quality care. They each spent several hours describing the activities of their days. All conversations and interviews were recorded and analyzed for common themes, and from this analysis the most common category of work identified was functional care. Assistants identified functional care as the "major contribution" to the overall health of residents and psychosocial care was identified as a close second contribution.[13]

Functional care descriptions include assistance with activities of daily living (ADL) such as bathing, toileting, and walking. The assistants described their work as promoting more independent functioning and maintaining health for the seniors in their care. They described meeting clients' needs with a combination of tasks and doing for residents what they could no longer do for themselves. A frequently described approach to maintaining or promoting functioning was to reduce ADLs to small, manageable tasks that residents could accomplish. These assistants also noted that they engaged in a variety of activities delegated to them by charge nurses. The most common tasks were taking vital signs such as blood pressure and pulse, but tasks also included taking temperatures and weights, measuring intake and output, noting percentage of meals eaten, and checking for and removing fecal impactions.

Home care assistants provide similar functional care as nursing home assistants. For instance, they help with activities of daily living such as bathing, dressing, eating, transferring, and toileting. They also perform some light housekeeping tasks. A home care assistant checks vital signs only if he or she is qualified as a health care assistant. One response from a home care assistant to the question, "So what exactly is it that you do?" provides a good descriptive picture. The assistant said, "If skilled medical services are the bricks of a house, home care services are the mortar." In other words, home care assistants provide the services that allow seniors to stay in their own homes for as long as possible.[14]

Functional care is typically very physical in nature and nursing homes have one of the highest rates of workplace injuries in the country. Nationally, there are 18.2 injuries per 100 workers in nursing homes, compared to 6.2 injuries among coal miners and 10.6 among construction workers.[15] Assistants routinely move and lift immobile individuals and sore backs were common complaints. Injuries are more frequent when nursing homes have insufficient staff. In home care, assistants routinely work alone—lifting and caring for their clients together—yet their injuries are frequently not reported.

Psychosocial Care

Psychosocial care considers a wide variety of interpersonal actions all influencing the emotional health of seniors, regardless of their cognitive levels. Assistants give psychosocial care at the same time as functional care, as well as throughout the day when the senior does not need immediate functional help. In the previously mentioned, 'expert assistants study' all assistants stated that their care centered on the senior's preferences and needs. For example, a bath is personalized and given according to a senior's preferences for more cold or hot water and a specific style of washing, as well as using preferred soaps (or no soap at all). Assistants emphasized residents' need to control their care as important to their emotional well-being. This was done by first encouraging residents to direct their assistants in their personal care. Then, gradually the assistants encouraged residents to physically become involved in their own care.

Another way to provide psychosocial care that assistants identified is through obtaining personal knowledge about residents by both encouraging residents to reminiscence about their personal interests and experiences, and by reading charts to learn their social histories and care needs. As one nursing assistant said, "You can come and talk to them and ask them about something that happened to them. They just kind of open up. Next time they see you, they will wave at you. And that makes me feel good when I do something like that"[16]

In some studies, nursing assistants felt they provided psychosocial care through their words of encouragement and comfort. Comments from one nursing home assistant reflect this:

> I feel like I have to be [good] to them in more ways than just getting
> them up and cleaning them up. They've got feelings like they are
> away from home. They are not able to do the things they once did
> and then they are brought into new surroundings . . . And I've got to
> be there for them, to soothe their minds and their bodies and make
> them feel this is a home away from home.[17]

A different way some assistants identified as supporting seniors' emotional needs was through supporting specific religious needs and general states of mind. Some assistants mentioned praying for their residents. One took a few of her residents to church. Several assistants felt the residents had a right to be moody and have bad days, and in that spirit, they endured hurtful comments on those days.

Nearly all observation studies noted that despite the enormous demands of physically needy and cognitively impaired residents, most assistants gave a great deal of sympathetic care. In fact, researchers were impressed with the commitment of the majority of assistants to the human dimensions of caring for seniors. The majority of assistants established positive relations with residents and were nearly always kind, with only an occasional mean remark. Furthermore, most of the time, the assistants did not get angry when dealing with difficult or abusive residents, and they often developed strategies to calm agitation.

In a home care study, assistants identified by their supervisors as "excellent" were interviewed about how they thought about their clients while doing work for them. Three common attitudes toward older clients were identified: patience, compassion, and respect. Several assistants said that by trying to imagine how seniors viewed things, they felt they understood their clients' needs and were more patient and respectful. Assistants also reminded themselves that their clients had once been like them—young, busy, active, and capable. They then treated the clients the way they themselves hoped to be treated as they aged. One home care assistant said, "Every day may be the last one for Mary. I keep this in mind and try to smile a lot and to hug. When I leave for the day, I want the feeling to be warm and friendly. I may be the last person that she ever sees."[18]

All "excellent" assistants stated that respect for older people was a basic tenet of their work. Although clients were dependent on workers for many services, workers still felt that they could learn and benefit from seniors' life experiences, an attitude which enhanced clients' self-esteem. One assistant said, "I try to treat my clients as if they were my parents. This is always in my mind."[19]

Custodial Care

Several observation studies reveal that psychosocial care can also be given in a negative manner, and such care is labeled custodial care. Custodial care is acting in a paternal manner, so the seniors' opinions are not considered—the opposite of good psychosocial care.

In the most comprehensive study of assistants' behaviors researchers first surveyed assistants regarding their views or stereotypes of older people and how they thought they treated their nursing home residents. For three months following this survey, researchers observed and recorded assistants' behaviors and facial expressions towards senior residents. Analysis of assistants' stereotypes, intentions, facial expressions, and behaviors revealed that those assistants less likely to stereotype older persons (either positively or negatively) exhibited more positive behaviors toward senior residents. Those who held negative stereotypes and who felt negative about their own aging were most likely to behave with impatience, anger, or irritation toward their senior residents, suggesting that deeply held stereotypes are the strongest predictors of behaviors.[20]

Another study, which attempted to identify personal values and how these influence care for seniors in nursing homes or assisted-living facilities, recorded all statements made by staff about residents.[21] After fifty hours of recording all comments were gathered and identified as positive or negative and as valuing autonomous or passive behaviors. Comments such as "she's real active or a real fighter" were coded as autonomy-valuing, while comments such as "never complains" and "behaving better" were coded as valuing passive behavior. After coding all comments, the researchers analyzed the origin and location of all comments. They found that not a single comment valuing autonomy in seniors came from assistants in nursing homes. Furthermore, approximately two-thirds of the negative comments from nursing assistants dealt with residents who interrupted daily routines and imposed "unreasonable demands." These comments clearly reinforced custodial care.

A study of attitudes toward mentally incompetent nursing home residents produced similar findings.[22] Researchers surveyed over 200 nursing home assistants about their attitudes towards their residents and beliefs about how to care for the mentally ill. Results indicated that nursing assistants have a fairly strong custodial orientation toward treatment of mental illness. The assistants with a higher level of custodial beliefs had greater general negativism toward seniors and lower levels of empathy. Also, the nursing assistants with negative attitudes toward the aged had less empathy towards their residents. Compared to nurses, assistants had the lowest empathy levels and the highest custodial orientations toward old people.

Mealtime Tasks

Meals are often one of the few activities seniors look forward to each day. Often, within the hour after seniors finish a meal, they start watching the clock for the next meal. Despite this eagerness, many seniors have eating and weight-maintenance problems. A primary task of assistants is, therefore, helping seniors with meals and fluid intake.

One observation study focused just on the mealtime assistance given by nursing assistants in nursing homes.[23] Twenty-nine nursing assistants were observed assisting with 60 meals provided to ten residents. All ten residents were functionally dependent, and eight were cognitively impaired. Observations of ineffective or negative assistance occurred much more than that of positive assistance. The most common negative action observed was the assistant assuming total control of what and how fast foods were consumed (95%). During only 5% of the meals did the assistant ask the resident if she or he wanted a particular food before offering it. One of the mealtime observations follows:

> A nursing assistant entered the dinning room and pulled up a chair to the table where a resident sat. Without greeting or even speaking to him, she picked up a spoon and began to feed him. He opened his mouth as each spoonful was offered. The nursing assistant watched as she fed him but never made eye contact.[24]

A few assistants exhibited positive meal assistance such as socializing with the resident during the meal, addressing the resident by name, and even sharing a meal with the resident. After observing a few of the nursing assistants trying to socialize with residents during the meal, the researcher noted that communicating with cognitively impaired persons seemed to take great skill and patience. Sharing a meal is one of the most basic human experiences, yet observations indicated that residents often ate their breakfasts alone in their rooms. Once, however, a nursing assistant was observed eating breakfast with a resident. The assistant got the resident up for breakfast and took her to the dining room so they could share a table. She brought toast and coffee from home for herself and ate it while she fed the resident. The nursing assistant said to the researcher, "No one likes to eat alone."[25]

Assistants in assisted-living facilities commented on how much better they liked meals in their facilities than in nursing homes. First, they mentioned that the seniors were easier to assist, as none needed actual help with their utensils. Still, many seniors needed foods identified or cut up prior to eating. Researchers also observed the assistants trying to make the meals more enjoyable with pleasant conversations and background music.

Efficient Work Styles

A working style is the way one organizes work tasks. Many assistants feel that an efficient style is of utmost importance if they are to stay on the job and not suffer burnout. Experienced assistants seem to have achieved an efficient style, while new assistants usually lack skill in organization and efficiency. To gain a greater understanding of nursing assistant work, one set of researchers spent five months working alongside and interviewing 30 nursing home assistants—15 who had worked less than three months, and 15 who had worked one year or more. The observations and comparisons of assistants' styles provide great insight into their daily challenges.[26]

Experienced assistants are able to integrate and complete multiple jobs simultaneously. One efficient assistant was observed assisting one resident to sit on the toilet while she helped the resident's roommate dress and filled the bathtub in the next room. Efficient, experienced assistants seemed to sequence their residents' care according to an unwritten, extremely efficient plan that got all jobs done within specific deadlines (usually by meals or bedtimes). This unwritten plan, unfortunately, did not permit assistants to meet residents' individual preferences. Assistants never asked seniors when they wanted various tasks done; they simply told them what tasks would be performed, and the seniors complied.

In contrast, novice assistants appeared more responsive to individual preferences and tended to respond to each request as it arose. For instance, if a new assistant was in the middle of a bed bath and a resident called out that she urgently needed to use the toilet, this assistant would cover the bathing resident and run help the distressed resident to the toilet. Experienced assistants typically sat residents on toilets before starting baths and then told the residents on the toilets to keep sitting and they would eventually feel an urge to go. As a consequence of the new assistants' style of responding to individual requests, other residents were often found half-bathed or sitting in bed for long time periods, waiting to get up and very angry with their "slow" assistant. Experienced assistants then were annoyed and would have to help finish the tasks of their inexperienced co-workers.

Observations in this study revealed that both new and experienced assistants sometimes cut quality care tasks, such as giving residents drinks or changing soiled clothes. When questioned, both the experienced and new assistants said these cuts were necessary to accomplish their routine work for the day (i.e., getting seniors out of bed, dressed, and fed). The researchers observed differences in how quality care tasks were cut. Experienced assistants seemed to make deliberate, preplanned cuts in their quality care tasks. These cuts could not be traced back to any one assistant, and it was often unclear if the task had been completed or not. An example of such a preplanned cut is not changing a wet diaper until the end of a shift; this may endanger the skin integrity of the incontinent resident, but an eventual decubitus ulcer could not be traced to any one assistant. The inexperienced assistants made quality care cuts too, but only as their deadlines or shift changes drew closer. In these instances, supervisors could clearly trace the undone tasks back to the inexperienced assistants. For instance, the new assistants may just not have time for their end of shift diaper changes, but have made all the other changes during their shift. Researchers labeled the new assistants as conducting "visible" quality cuts, while the experienced assistants made "invisible" cuts.

In another work style study, a researcher worked as an assistant for over a year to identify assistants' methods of enhancing efficiency by informal or "hidden" work.[27] She found that assistants did many things to improve their efficiency, some of which involved teamwork and others which involved competition. One example of teamwork occurred during meal preparations when one assistant poured the beverages for all residents while another passed out the bibs or napkins. An example of competitive efficiency was seen in the everyday silent race to reach the easy feeders, or residents who could eat fast and did not tend to choke or drool. Another efficient work method was the memorization of residents' personal habits and preferences. Assistants quickly fulfilled these preferences without wasting time or words, such as quickly putting the correct number of sugar packets in coffee cups when dropping off the meal tray.

Another observation study noted assistants' responses to proposed improvements to client care that interfered with their established work styles.[28] For eight months researchers observed and took notes on nursing assistants' responses to a proposed new toileting program to decrease incontinence. The assistants were quite resistant to the program, and several interviews identified their reasons. The primary reason seemed to be that changes were interpreted as challenging their efficiency and knowledge. A typical comment was, "It just doesn't feel right to toilet a resident farther down the hall, and it takes me more steps and time."[29] Another reason identified from conversations, but not directly stated, was that the assistants often didn't appreciate the importance of new programs: "Things were fine the way they had arranged them, so why change things?"[30]

Home care assistants' efficient work styles do not seem as well documented. Nonetheless, some home care studies have involved interviews of home care assistants regarding how to do their work more effectively. Researchers observed and interviewed assistants from five different home care agencies over a six-month period.[31] These researchers found that nearly all tasks were carried out alone by the assistants. A select few tasks were carried out by two assistants due to the senior's weight or unwillingness to cooperate. The majority of these tasks involved providing direct care. The remaining tasks were making a bed or moving furniture for cleaning. The direct care tasks rated as most stressful for home care assistants were lifting seniors up in bed and putting on anti-embolism stockings. The most stressful non-patient-handling tasks were cranking up the bed, moving furniture, and making the bed.

Assistants listed over 600 factors contributing to stress. They were further grouped into categories of body mechanics, patient factors, and environmental factors. Body mechanics were actions such as bending, reaching, and lifting away from the body. Patient factors were weight, inability to help, resistance, combativeness, and cognitive deficits. Environmental factors included beds that were too low, nonadjustable, nonmoveable from the wall, too wide, and not electric.

Devices the assistants used included mechanical lifts, gait belts, hair washing trays for use with residents in bed, and hand-held shower hoses. Seniors sometimes had purchased or rented mechanical lifts that were used for transfers in and out of bed, on and off the toilet, and in and out of chairs. Gait belts were used for these same tasks. Assistants' ideas for reducing stress included knowledge of body mechanics to be more careful; keeping the patient close to self while lifting; giving the senior medication for combativeness and spasticity; and having the senior help more. Environmental factors included assistants using adjustable beds; seniors wearing nonrestrictive clothing; and having assistive devices for lifting and transferring seniors. Recommendations for policy changes from assistants were to permit more than one assistant for heavy and difficult clients and to allow more time for each home visit. The assistants identified the following approaches as being most helpful: having beds that adjust for various positions; not using double or water beds; putting regular beds up on blocks; and arranging beds so that assistant can work from both sides of the bed.

Extra Initiatives

Extra initiatives are the activities assistants do over and above tasks that are required. Supervisors sometimes note these extra initiatives and sometimes family members note them, but always the assistants feel that their seniors appreciate the extra care. Researchers first recognized extra initiatives in nursing home studies when many assistants seemed to take pride in their residents' appearances. They saw assistants taking the time to put attractive clothing, make-up, and jewelry on seniors when such activities were not necessary. Other extra activities noted were how some assistants kept residents' rooms well organized and clean and took pride in their ability to cajole reluctant residents to eat. Researchers noted that assistants completed all these activities without any prompting from supervisors or family members.[32]

In describing their work, some nursing home assistants mentioned that they try to distract residents from loneliness or depression with diversions such as food treats and surprises. These assistants often provided gifts and individualized services according to residents' requests or needs. Several assistants regularly used their own time to shop for requested items—"little things like Vaseline or powder." [33] These assistants also tried to keep residents' rooms attractive and pleasing according to their specific preferences. Each assistant mentioned trying to be aware of and reduce minor annoyances to residents.

Another area of extra initiatives noted is in the clinical care arena. One study found that the nursing home assistants labeled as excellent were often performing clinical tasks before their charge nurses requested them. In interviews with the nurses, one charge nurse described her most expert nursing assistant by saying, "She assumes responsibility for initiating care, especially when the charge nurse is not available."[34] The researchers noted that most extra activities were not performed under direct supervision, but that assistants notified charge nurses of the outcomes (actual blood pressure readings, weights, etc.) One assistant described her extra initiative this way:

> ... You see something on the leg; maybe they bumped it or fell during the night. . . . You report it to the nurse and see if she's seen it. If she has, you're going to ask her, "What are we going to do for it? Do you want me to do it or are you going to take care of it?"[35]

Home care assistants provide different types of extra initiatives. Interviews with these assistants reveal that they like to think of their extra care as "turning a difficult home situation into a personal challenge"[36] for them to overcome. One home care assistant said, "The client I had before used to beat his wife. I would run in front of her and get him to stop."[37] Another assistant said, "I once had a Romanian client who didn't speak English. When I didn't understand her, she had tantrums and would throw things. I would sit down and pray. I tried to stay calm. After a while, we had no problems."[38]

Another home care assistant felt strongly that a stimulating environment was important for increasing her clients' alertness and connections to the outside world. She said that when she felt an apartment contributed to a client's negative condition, she used her camera to take pictures of the entire apartment. She then brought the pictures to her agency, which put the client on a list for a safe, comfortable place. She stated she had helped quite a few clients move to nicer places![39] Several home care assistants would bring puzzles and cards to stimulate their clients until they started talking more, while yet another assistant asked her client's daughter to buy her a radio. At first, they just listened to music together. Then they started to listen to and discuss the news together. Now the client listens to the news in the early morning and starts telling the assistant about it when she arrives.[40] These home care assistants received great satisfaction from helping to improve situations for their clients.

Abusive Activities

One last area, abuse of seniors including ignoring their feelings or needs, is considered from the frontline staff perspective. Two studies involved interviews with nursing home assistants about witnessing resident abuse (either by other assistants or by themselves). Both studies found that assistants saw much more psychological than physical abuse. The first survey found that 36% of nursing assistants had witnessed at least one incident of physical abuse in the preceding year, while 81% had observed at least one incident of psychological abuse in the preceding year.[41] The most frequent type of psychological abuse involved yelling at a resident, and the most common physical abuse was restraining, followed by pushing, grabbing, shoving, or pinching.

A second study found that over 90% of assistants had seen or heard of residents being abused, either physically or emotionally.[42] Most episodes were verbal and consisted of yelling or saying mean things to residents. One assistant reported another assistant as saying, "Remember, you need me, but I don't need you. Don't forget it."[43] The assistants also witnessed neglect ranging from ignoring call lights to telling residents to use their diapers instead of getting a bedpan. Physical abuse was usually not directly witnessed but evidenced by bruises or marks on seniors the next day. Many assistants claimed residents were right in not reporting their abuse as they might suffer possible retribution.

Studies of nursing assistants who are burned out reveal that many of their behaviors were actually psychologically abusive towards the seniors they were caring for. For instance, the assistants who admitted to being burned out stated that they got to the point of just giving physical help without speaking to the senior. Researchers noted the behavior of these assistants as sullen and unresponsive as well as engaging in regularly ignoring calls for help. An example of this behavior was observed with a demented senior in a nursing home. Assistants brought a resident back to his floor from the dining room because his pants had accidentally been drenched by a coffee spill. He waited in his wheelchair by the nursing station to be changed, extremely confused and continually asking for help, but none of the assistants who passed acknowledged him. In fact, the assistants were observed as avoiding eye contact with him. After half an hour, a charge nurse asked an assistant to help him.[44]

Other negative behaviors observed by burned out assistants were taunting and teasing, cold stares, speaking in gruff voices, and making cruel remarks. In one case of taunting, three assistants in an elevator with an alert wheelchair-bound resident loudly laughed among themselves about how bad he smelled. One assistant said, "He needs a fire hose to clean him down."[45]

Researchers who observed these behaviors found that most assistants did some negative behaviors only on an occasional basis, and that these behaviors were primarily treating residents with indifference and apathy. For example, one assistant changed residents' beds in a hurried, distracted way, barely talking to seniors and muttering to herself about how tired she was. She practically threw a shirt on one senior, not even noticing that it was wrinkled, torn, and the wrong size.[46] This erratic behavior was often blamed on physical exhaustion or burnout on the part of the assistant and fortunately, the majority of assistants observed engaged in this behavior only at their lowest times.

Values and Satisfactions

When nursing assistants feel satisfied and are working in an organization that recognizes and respects their personal values, they are happier themselves and demonstrate empathy and compassion more easily to seniors. Satisfied assistants tend to help others more, complain less, and give extra effort toward doing their jobs. One's values are desirable, often unconscious personal characteristics that powerfully influence behaviors. By exploring what is valued by nursing assistants, working conditions can be improved.

Job satisfaction dimensions are a more definable area than are personal values for nursing assistants. A person can be satisfied with some aspects of a job but not with others. Yet, in addition to rating how satisfied he or she is with a job dimension, it is important also to rate how important that job dimension is to the person. In other words, some job areas may be very important and unsatisfactory (e.g., salary), while others may be just somewhat important and very satisfactory.

After reviewing many studies, nursing assistants seem to share one common personal value (ambition) and two job satisfaction dimensions (offering valued services and interpersonal relationships). In addition, home care assistants have one unique job dimension giving them much satisfaction (autonomy).

Ambition

The majority of nursing home assistants identified ambition as having an underlying power and importance in their daily lives. From a list of ten values, over 100 nursing home assistants selected this value as most important in their own lives. [47] Ambition was defined as being hardworking and aspiring. Above all other values, nursing assistants viewed themselves as having ambition both in their personal lives and at work. Another study of nursing assistants found that "hard work" was identified as one of their top attributes. [48] In both these studies, other values assistants thought appropriate for describing themselves were being helpful, cheerful, and capable. However, claimed most frequently was this one value—ambition or hard work—as the assistants proudly discussed all they did to survive and support their families.

These studies entailed very direct questions; a completely different style of study using conversations and observations of assistants found they consistently emulated the values of ambition and hard work. [49] The researchers found nursing assistants as commonly living on the edge of financial survival with little, if any, physical or psychological support and working full time, often in more than one job. Most had endured severe personal conflicts such as living in alcoholic families, flight from war-torn countries, or domestic violence. The assistants had triumphed over their personal circumstances and were currently providing as stable a life as possible for themselves and their families.

Based on their responses to interviews, researchers divided assistants into two categories. Those who believed that they or their family members would have better lives if they just kept working were labeled "strivers," while those who were just trying to hold onto the most stable life they could and were cynical about a brighter future were labeled "endurers." Although categorizing people is a distasteful action, a review of this work reveals that despite their labels as strivers or endurers, all assistants demonstrated real ambition within their personal lives. Seeing and hearing the personal odds many nursing assistants have overcome and then their current daily struggles put the value of "ambition" in an understandable framework. Listening to both staff histories and their interpretations of their lives greatly enhanced our understanding of essential frontline staff.

Valuable Services

Job satisfaction ratings of nursing assistants compared to those in jobs paying equivalent wages are much higher in the dimensions of "job significance" and "seeing outcomes from their work."[50] Study after study reveals that the majority of assistants get great satisfaction from helping others. For instance, one nursing home assistant said, "I could go down the street and get a job at Burger King, but I care about these residents. If I weren't here, they would be much worse off."[51] The ability to help people and do meaningful work is an extremely satisfying element of assistants' work. This high level of satisfaction is found across the spectrum of assistants working in low income urban areas, in rural areas, and in more affluent suburbs.[52]

Home care assistants identify the same sense of contributing valuable services that nursing home assistants do. They feel a sense of accomplishment in the work they do and like seeing the visible results of their efforts (a senior surviving in her or his home). Furthermore, they truly believe their work is valuable both to the individual senior and to society.[53] One home health care assistant explained that her primary goal was to help seniors through a crisis or acute episode, and bring them to their maximum level of independence. After this, she explained that a home care assistant provides valuable services that may make the difference between seniors staying healthy and going into the hospital. Also, assisting seniors with light housekeeping, nutrition, and reminders to take medications consistently may make a significant improvement in seniors' quality of life.[54]

To better understand assistants' typical concerns, one researcher worked as an assistant for two years in four different nursing homes analyzing everyday conversations.[55] He found that everyday talk centered on not having enough money for rent, transportation, or children's necessities. In one of these conversations, the researcher asked assistants why they did not seek better paying jobs. The assistants considered this an insult. After several silent minutes, one older nursing assistant, looking indignant and angry, said, "This is what I *do*."[56] Clearly, her profession was something she had practiced for 14 years, and it included her own valuable skills and knowledge. Being a nursing assistant was valued as a great contribution to society's elderly population, one she was proud to perform. As another nursing assistant said, "There aren't that many jobs where you can get eight 'thank-yous' in a day. I get a paycheck every day and a stipend every two weeks."[57]

Interpersonal Relationships

Most nursing assistants hold high expectations for positive relationships with their clients. In fact, 95% of assistants expect to be like family to their seniors.[58] These assistants see themselves as nurturing and compassionate toward their clients. They notice when their senior clients are troubled or worried, and encourage them to talk about their feelings. These assistants report that they expect and most often enjoy close relationships with their aging clients. In fact, these relationships provide some of the strongest motivators for assistants of any type of long-term care organization to stay at their jobs. One study of nursing assistants asked the question, "What would you change if you could change anything at the facility?" The nursing assistants all suggested special things the residents needed. This response reveals the love and sensitive awareness that these assistants had for their residents.[59]

A two-year study of nursing assistants found that when questioned about quality of care, assistants focused primarily on the quality of the relationship between the seniors and staff, and how care was delivered.[60] Assistants deemed relationships as the central determinant of both quality of care and quality of life. The nursing assistants believed that high quality care meant developing relationships with residents and then using those relationships to enhance the quality of residents' lives. The assistants provided many examples of building their relationships and reported that nurturing these relationships improved both the quality of care for seniors and the quality of the job experience for themselves. Several nursing assistants stated they enjoyed listening to the residents, hearing their histories and learning from their knowledge.[61]

Great interpersonal relationships are found among home care assistants, just as they are among nursing home assistants.[62] Researchers conducted interviews with over 400 home care assistants regarding their relationships with their clients. Assistants overwhelmingly reported enjoying special relationships with their clients, and in many cases, the assistants felt almost like surrogate family members. Again, the majority of nursing assistants derived great satisfaction from their work and enjoyed close relationships with their clients. They considered the ability to develop close interpersonal relationships with their clients as one of the most rewarding aspects of their work.

In a different home care study, many assistants gave their seniors caring telephone calls, sent special occasion cards, or gave small gifts.[63] Furthermore, when interviewers asked the assistants how they suspected their senior clients felt about them, they seemed very reflective. The majority believed that their senior clients displayed higher levels of affection for them, and felt that the seniors really cared about them as individuals, often thinking about them long after they had left their homes.

Autonomy

Home care assistants are just as motivated by the sense of doing valued work and developing relationships with seniors as nursing home assistants, but they identified one additional job satisfaction area: the autonomy to decide how to perform work and set one's own pace.[64] In several surveys, home care assistants mentioned their sense of doing valuable work and their autonomy as the best parts of their jobs. This last value then needs to be recognized as a contributor to home care assistants' overall job satisfaction.[65]

There is no doubt that specific values and job dimensions are personal and organizational motivators for assistants. Long-term care administrators and nurses need to be aware of these areas and recognize and respect them. For as many assistants stated, they complete their work in spite of the money and many unsatisfactory job dimensions. In other words, assistants complete this work for the internal rewards of helping human kind in their greatest time of need.

Dissatisfactions and Challenges

Extremely high turnover rates among long-term care assistants are one sign of persistent job dissatisfaction. National surveys reveal that turnover is a long-standing problem that does not seem to be improving. In the latest annual survey, nursing assistants' turnover rates exceeded 60% in 32 states, and 100% in 10 states.[66] To deal with these high turnover numbers, administrators are forced to demand more time from their current staff. One study found that over three-fourth of assistants had been asked to change their scheduled shifts, to stay late, or to come in early in the previous two months.[67] To add to this challenge, our aging population is growing, and the U.S. Bureau of Labor Statistics predicts that the number of nursing assistants needs to increase by 39% in the next ten years.[68] In light of these numbers, administrators are challenged and pressured to address dissatisfactions among their staff.

Another reason for administrators to be concerned with frontline staff challenges is that assistants with low job satisfaction can be very demoralizing to the seniors receiving care and services. Nearly all areas of staff dissatisfaction eventually impacts seniors.[69] In other words, low job satisfaction is linked not only to assistants leaving their jobs, but also with poor job performance. Surprisingly, the areas of lowest satisfaction have not changed for over a decade: low pay and benefits, problematic management and supervisor styles, overwhelming workloads, and hearing accusations or complaints versus praise.[70] Not surprisingly, these challenges have led to a high percentage of assistants feeling exhaustion and burnout.[71] Five of the most common dissatisfactions are reviewed here:

Financial Security

Wages and lack of benefits are areas of dissatisfaction among nearly all nursing home assistants. Compared to similarly educated, hourly wage workers, nursing assistants have the lowest satisfaction ratings for pay and benefits. In all surveys of this area, nearly all nursing assistants were moderately to strongly dissatisfied with their pay, and, as previously stated, many assistants worked extra shifts or second jobs to "cover basics."[72] One nursing home assistant stated, "As a nurse's aide, I know from experience we are underpaid, under-staffed, and overworked. There are no benefits and the medical insurance costs more than I make in one month!"[73]

Adequate health insurance is another area of concern regarding financial security. A study of U.S. labor statistics in the late 1990's found that among occupation groups, assistants had the highest rates of uninsured workers and accounted for 37% of uninsured health care personnel. Coverage varied by place of employment with 20% of nursing home assistants uninsured, compared with 16% of assistants in other health care areas. Unionized assistants had a higher rate of insurance than did non-unionized assistants. Overall, it was found that assistants were losing health coverage more rapidly than other Americans were, and they were providing care that they and their children could not expect to receive.[74]

Home care assistants' low wages are also very unsatisfactory. In addition to dissatisfaction with low hourly wages and lack of benefits, the assistants are also unhappy with their lack of guaranteed hours per week due to the scheduling and reimbursement system most agencies use. Assistants are assigned clients and then paid for the hours negotiated for the visits. If an assigned client goes to the hospital or visits a relative, the assistant is out those paid hours until the client returns home or the agency assigns him or her another client. One home care assistant said,

> The best benefit package I ever had was at a hospital. At the home care agency we have no benefits, you have no mileage, you are running your car to the ground. You don't get paid in between visits. If you visit at one home for two hours and need to travel to another home you are paid only for the time spent with a patient. Not on the road.[75]

A survey of home care assistants in Washington found that nearly half did not have health insurance, sick leave, or vacation days.[76] This situation is similar in other states, with a national survey finding that over 70% of home health assistants are able to secure only part time work, forcing them to juggle two or more jobs simultaneously with different employers.[77] Many agencies (urban or rural) rely heavily on government contracts. These agencies are considered vendors to the state and pay their employees the state-stipulated wages—usually minimum wage, without benefits. In South Dakota, when the state changed its system from state-employed home care assistants to vendors, former state employees switched to working for independent home care agency vendors, and their hourly wages went down by $1.00 per hour as they continued to care for the same clients. This low pay is similar in other states, as states often stipulate minimum wages for their vendors but usually do not stipulate benefits. Hence, the majority of home care workers do not have guaranteed hours, health insurance, or pensions.

Despite unhappiness with low wages, this area of dissatisfaction is not consistently correlated with overall job dissatisfaction or even with high turnover rates. Some studies have found a connection, while others have not. This lack of a consistent association may be due to individual needs. One study found that if over 75% of an assistant's salary went to essentials (shelter and food), then he or she should strongly consider different work. For the majority of assistants, low wages and benefits were not the primary reasons for seeking different employment but were significant contributing factors. As one assistant who left the profession said, "I make more money cleaning offices, emptying trash and wiping down exam tables and sinks and mopping floors, than I did taking care of the elderly. And that is a damn shame."[78]

One study presented very troubling, yet realistic questions at the end of their report. "Can an uninsured health aide with limited access to care for back pain, seizures or a cough safely lift and feed frail patients? Can those denied health coverage and care for themselves and their children be expected to care compassionately for strangers?"[79]

This issue is getting worse, not better. The problems in assisted-living facilities are beginning to look similar to those in the nursing home industry. Turnover rates are about the same or lower than that found in nursing homes and hourly wages are also slightly lower.[80]

Supervisors & Management

Many nursing assistants identify their supervisors and general management as their strongest points of dissatisfaction. In fact, poor supervisory relations are the most common reason given by assistants for leaving their jobs. Several studies found that supervisors and administrators are much more responsible for assistants leaving their jobs than either low wages or lack of benefits. Assistants described supervisor dissatisfaction with a variety of phrases, but in general, feelings of support and trust were absent. One assistant in a focus group said, "I never had a job that was more battering to self-esteem than assistant work. I don't mean patient-wise, I am talking management; it is a killer."[81] One national survey reported that from 71 to 84% of nursing home assistants did not think they could rely on their supervisors when things got tough, did not feel their supervisors were willing to listen to their job problems, and did not think supervisors or administrators respected them.[82]

In a different survey, more than half of the assistants were dissatisfied with the lack of feedback they received from their supervisors and with the lack of attention the supervisors gave to the assistants' suggestions and opinions. Furthermore, two-thirds of assistants reported that their supervisors hardly ever let them know how helpful they had been or recognized them for good work.[83] Other surveys reveal that nursing assistants feel their supervisors do not encourage them to use their skills to their fullest and do not treat them as equal members of the health care team. The words of one nursing assistant illustrate these feelings:

> Many nurses and LPNs don't like "stepping down" to do an aide's job. They say, 'I didn't go to school to do patient care.' They become good at giving orders. Nurses who do help are sometimes told, 'You're being too nice to aides; that's not what you were hired for.' Many don't have the foggiest idea what we do. They issue unreasonable, ludicrous orders and make promises to residents and fami-

lies that can't be kept. This causes chaos. And God forbid if you
question the head nurse.[84]

The most common complaints found in nearly all surveys were little or no
feedback and lack of recognition for good work from management or supervisors. In one study, only one of twelve assistants interviewed stated that she felt
respected by her superiors. One assistant reported that in the absence of respect
from supervisors, she would find some consolation within herself, knowing she
had done a good job.[85]

Another area of dissatisfaction is instructions from high-pressured supervisors, which puts the assistant in an awkward position such as being expected to
falsify records. One nursing home assistant explained, "I couldn't give showers
because I had too many 'total care' patients to take care of. So my supervisor
told me to write it down anyway because the state might be coming and she had
to show that it was done."[86] This practice was acknowledged by supervisors as
common in their industry as a necessary practice to deal with demanding regulations.

Assistants often discussed negative impressions of management at the same
time as supervisors. Just as poor relations with supervisors is significant, so is
"bad management" given as a reason for leaving the job. Additionally, poor administrator relations lead to poor institutional loyalty and increases assistants'
intentions to look for employment elsewhere. Several studies with undercover
researchers posing as nursing assistants noted very tense relationships between
management and labor in nursing homes. Several times administrators used in-
timidation tactics against these undercover researchers thinking they were nursing assistants.[87]

The absence of respect or appreciation for quality work greatly contributes
to assistants' job dissatisfaction and turnover.[88] In nursing homes with high
turnover rates, assistants often claimed they felt demeaned by administrators and
were treated as if they had no common sense or work ethics. Several complained
that they had no one to talk with about job problems or that their supervisors did
not seem concerned when they did share problems.[89] In one national survey,
over half of nursing assistants claimed to never or only minimally be involved in
care planning conferences and 75% of nursing assistants were rarely or never
involved in residents' pre-admission conferences.[90] Nursing assistants felt their
absence from these meetings indicated a lack of respect for their opinions and
claimed this treatment was related to their organization's high turnover.

Home care assistants seemed just as dissatisfied as nursing home assistants
in these areas. Many complained of lack of participation in their clients' care
plans and lack of supportive supervisors. These areas were also found to be related to general job dissatisfaction. Not being able to talk to their supervisors or
their supervisors ignoring their comments were common complaints.[91]

Interestingly, good relationships with supervisors and managers seem to be
just as influential as negative ones. In nursing homes with positive perceptions
of managers and supervisors, the assistants tend to have significantly less turnover. At one facility noted for its positive leadership, one assistant's response to
being asked if she would work somewhere else for a dollar more an hour was,

"Would I leave my family for a dollar an hour?"[92] Tokens of appreciation mentioned by nursing home assistants include paying for meals when they worked overtime, recognizing overtime assistants in monthly newsletters and Christmas gifts or bonuses.[93]

Assistants in assisted-living facilities seem more satisfied with their supervisors. In a national survey, assistants gave their employers high marks for hiring competent supervisors.[94] This is good news, especially in light of the insufficient pay these assistants received.

Workloads and Staffing Ratios

Staffing ratios and workloads go hand in hand. A staff ratio is the number of clients assigned to one staff person (e.g., 15:1); the larger the ratio, the heavier the workload. Another way to measure workload is the number of hours per day an assistant can give each senior. Several national organizations recommend about 4.1 hours of skilled care per day, but this is far from the amount currently given in most nursing homes.

Workload or staff ratios in long-term care facilities are widely discussed as an unsatisfactory job dimension by nearly all institutional staff. The number of nursing home seniors assigned to assistants was a subject of constant conflict. Most private-pay nursing homes assign fewer residents to their assistants than Medicaid nursing homes (nursing homes accepting large percentages of Medicaid clients) which typically assign day shift assistants 12 to 18 residents each. One study of proprietary nursing homes in the South found the number of residents assigned to an assistant ranged from 6 to 36. However, the highest numbers were usually for assistants on night shifts or on units with ambulatory residents capable of some self care.

This area of frustration and stress is one with which the assistants learned to cope creatively. Unfortunately, their coping methods often come at the price of additional stress and lower quality care for seniors. One assistant with 13 residents admitted she rarely finished her work and often went home feeling bad about what she had not done. Several assistants admitted that they had not been able to care for their large caseloads when they had been new, but that they had gradually learned the tricks or skills to manage. One assistant on the evening shift admitted she felt okay with 15 residents because most were in bed by 7:30 anyway. Some night shift assistants noted that they worked in pairs and that the work went much more efficiently. Several assistants stated they knew they could not give residents much attention with their heavy workloads, but they tried to anyway. A night duty assistant said her workload was not bad except that the residents loved to talk. She figured out she could give each resident 15 minutes, but that was all or she would get behind.[95]

Workload dissatisfaction and poor managerial relations go hand in hand, as assistants often voiced the feeling that administrators were not hiring enough staff. Many assistants felt administrators just did not want to pay for more staff, and they felt that they could not provide good care when the administrators had assigned them too many clients. Nursing assistants stated they wanted to take pride in the nursing home they were working in and often felt administrators were not responsive enough to seniors by keeping the staffing low. Some assistants described the poor staff-to-client ratios as "deliberate understaffing." These feelings may have some validity, as a recent government study found that as spending per resident day increased, the proportion of spending devoted to nursing care declined.[96]

One two-year study with researchers observing and interviewing assistants found that when short staffed, the assistants had a number of "time saving measures."[97] Seniors were not given the time to choose what they wanted to wear; were not allowed to wear favorite clothing that took time to put on or take off; grooming preferences like braids and makeup were not addressed; oral care, walking, and range of motion exercises were eliminated; and even bathing tasks were shortened to just the "faces and bottoms." Visibility and potential accountability influenced how the assistants cut corners. For example, assistants were more likely to pick up dirty linen on a hallway floor than clean up a senior who was lying in a urine soaked bed. Toileting tasks were found to be one of the first activities to go when short staffed. The assistants described how despite knowing this was important they just could not do it and recognized that seniors who had once been continent were now incontinent because they made them wait too long for help to the toilet. Not surprisingly, the assistants did not report to their supervisors that toileting was not done, as they knew this was unacceptable. They explained that the impossibility of following the toileting plan when so short staffed must be obvious to supervisors, so why discuss it.

One study found that staff who described their nursing homes as providing high quality care worked there twice as long as those who felt the care was poor.[98] Another study found that assistants initially sought work because they liked helping and working with people, and they continued to enjoy this aspect of their work. Yet, overwhelmingly, they emphasized that they did not like to work when short staffed, seeing residents given less than optimum care.[99]

Indignities & Abuse

Just as abusive activities towards seniors have been recognized, abuse (primarily psychological abuse) towards assistants is also recognized. During interviews and conversations, many nursing home assistants voiced dissatisfaction with clients' family members' lack of respect for them. Several assistants voiced the feeling that family members assumed they neglected their relatives and their work. Assistants wanted family members to know that they were doing their best under heavy workloads. One assistant said, "Please understand I take care of eight to ten other residents and try to cooperate instead of making unrealistic demands."[100] In addition to doing their best physically, the assistants wanted family members to know that they truly cared about their relatives and often loved them. Furthermore, because residents often tell assistants things they do not tell their families, families need to treat assistants with respect and consider their opinions.

For home care assistants, dissatisfaction centered on family members asking them to do things that were not part of their jobs. Assistants reported being expected to do family laundry or other housecleaning chores for the entire family.

Such unpleasant experiences, most commonly being treated as a maid, were reported by less than 20% of home care assistants,[101] while 14% had families ask them to do things that were not part of their jobs. One assistant reported finding a sink full of the family's dirty dishes upon her arrival one morning. She carefully washed one place setting and used it for her client's breakfast and for every meal that day.

Another indignity experienced by nearly all assistants at some point is being hurt by agitated or demented seniors.[102] Physical insults were primarily experienced as the senior kicking, slapping, scratching, or biting. Many assistants reported that seniors with aggressive tendencies were "especially dangerous" when they were being dressed or bathed. Home care assistants reported more verbal insults, such as being yelled at or belittled.

Nursing assistants at all types of facilities and home care agencies reported hearing or being the target of racial remarks by seniors and family members. Dark-skinned assistants reported comments and behaviors from seniors about not wanting their dark hands to touch them. Some also made hurtful comments such as "the only thing that those blacks are good for is stealing." Nevertheless, residents and family members were not the only ones to make such remarks, administrators were heard making racial comments, too.[103]

In summary, although many assistants were reluctant to talk, psychological insults truly bothered them and when pushed to talk, some assistants shared their experiences. In one study, nearly half of the nursing home assistants reported they had received accusations from residents and their family members of inadequate care or theft.[104] Nearly one-third reported that residents had insulted them or made racial slurs against them. Also, several assistants said family members questioned them about their relative's care in a tone implying neglect or incompetence. Many assistants reported that while these behaviors and comments hurt, they understood that they could not hold many of the seniors responsible. On the other hand, comments from family members did bother them.

Inadequate Training

There is little consensus regarding how much training assistants should receive, but nearly all assistants claim they want more. Training for assistants, where mandated, is usually short (75 to 100 hours, depending on the state) and often inadequate to help assistants succeed at their demanding jobs. As previously stated, many assistants (home care and assisted-living assistants) receive no formal training at all. Despite receiving or not receiving original training, few opportunities are available for skill upgrading or advancement. Many feel this limits the ability of assistants to have a career path or long term success as a nursing assistant.[105]

A national survey of assisted-living assistants found distressing perceptions. The majority of assistants claimed to be adequately trained, yet when answering questions regarding normal aging and appropriate actions to take for various ailments, it was clear they were not knowledgeable. In fact, they demonstrated little correct knowledge of aging.[106]

The assistants want to feel confident that they are doing a job correctly. In focus groups of home care assistants, the assistants cited orientation and training as the number one issue affecting their retention, and the researchers noted that many workers left their jobs within days of starting because they did not feel prepared for the work.[107] In one nursing home study, 65% of assistants identified more training as a way their job could be improved. Similarly, assistants considering employment in home care agencies identified "educational opportunities" and "good orientation programs" as very important in selecting their next employer. Training or in-services were repeatedly mentioned as a way jobs could be improved by both home care and nursing home assistants.[108, 109, 110]

Specific topics about which assistants want more information include how to deal with tempers and aggressive behaviors and communication and problem-solving with residents and family members.[111, 112] Other topic areas for desired training are interpersonal skills with clients and co-workers, as well as understanding and managing persons with cognitive impairments.[113, 114]

Burnout

When dissatisfactions accumulate and are ignored, the logical progression is to a state of burnout. Burned out staff not only can injure themselves, but also have a high probability of injuring the very seniors they are trying to serve. Burnout has many definitions, but the simplest is: "a state of chronic dissatisfaction resulting in minimal commitment to the job."[115] Burned out staff usually want to quit, but for a variety of reasons do not. In burnout, dissatisfactions gradually overwhelm the staff member and result in psychological withdrawal. The most common components of burnout are emotional exhaustion, depersonalization, and a feeling of lack of accomplishment. Studies measuring burnout found that many nursing home assistants experience moderate to high levels of emotional exhaustion and depersonalization. Researchers found these assistants frequently to feel emotionally exhausted from their work and that they admitted to depersonalizing the seniors they cared for by providing physical help without recognition of residents' humanity.[116, 117] Examples of burnout behavior were reported in the abusive activities section; please refer back for more information.

Conclusion

Across the country, the long-term care industry is experiencing the highest rates of vacancies and turnover of assistants in its history. It seems as if the industry presumed an endless supply of low income women willing to work as assistants—always available to provide care despite job conditions and wages that kept them dissatisfied and among the working poor. With our growing senior population the best administrators must have an ability to attract frontline assistants within an increasingly competitive environment. Furthermore, in order to provide high quality care, they must ensure a respectful caring work environment. Nursing assistants' needs are consistent from year to year; financial security of a "living wage" with health insurance and full employment, safe or decent workloads, better training and in-service opportunities, support from supervisors, and respect for them as significant human beings.[118]

The late Mark Jerstad, former CEO of the Evangelical Lutheran Good Samaritan Society, went through the mandated training to become a nursing assistant after becoming a CEO. This experience, he said, was a humbling reminder of just how easily we can get out of touch with the daily reality of caregiving.[119] Now every nursing home administrator in his organization is required to spend one day a year working side-by-side with a nursing assistant. This is an excellent start toward enhancing understanding of the backbone and heart of an organization, but it is not enough.

There is more to learn than is possible from a one day shadowing experience with a nursing assistant. The stress of surviving on a low income, with lack of essential securities such as health insurance and sick days, greatly influences the lives of frontline assistants and how they are able to work. This background mixed with feeling disrespected by employers can negatively impact assistants' behaviors in caregiving.

Frontline assistants seem genuinely to love helping people and find this is one of their greatest job satisfactions. Administrators can enhance their skills in providing a nurturing environment by listening to the complete voices and perspectives of their frontline attendants. Hearing about their home lives, which impact their capacity for caring, and learning about their experience of overall workloads and daily challenges—as well as the behaviors that are hidden from outsiders—can help administrators know and address assistants' concerns more effectively. Direct care assistants have a critical role to play in improving the quality of long-term care services. To make the most of their ideas and creativity, they must make their voices heard and administrators must be listening.

CR80

Discussion Questions

1   Compare the job tasks for frontline staff in home care agencies, assisted-living facilities and nursing homes. Identify where the tasks are similar and where they are unique for each frontline position.

2. Discuss the personal challenges and personal satisfactions that each frontline staff position provides.

3. How can having experience as one type of assistant benefit a person when moving to another type of assistant position? Are there possible disadvantages of moving from one type of frontline staff position to another? What are these potential disadvantages?

4. Nearly 90% of frontline staff members are women with few support systems. Many of these workers are unmarried heads of household with dependent children and low incomes. In addition, a large percentage of them are from ethnic minorities. What life experience skills could these workers use in their daily work with seniors?

5. Five primary functions were identified that most frontline staff perform: functional care; psychosocial care (in contrast to custodial care); nourishment tasks; efficient work style activities; and extra initiatives (versus abusive activities). Describe these functions in your own words. Give two examples of each function, one which is a positive experience for seniors and the other which is a negative experience for seniors.

6. Describe custodial care. Can an assistant provide "good" custodial care? List practical methods used in order to identify when staff are providing custodial care. How should administrators deal with staff members who often provide custodial care?

7. Describe the differences between mealtimes at nursing homes versus assisted-living facilities. How can mealtimes be turned into positive interactions without breaking the nursing home's budget?

8. Both experienced and new frontline staff members say that quality care cuts are necessary to accomplish routine work each day. Some make "invisible" cuts, while others just partake in visible cuts. Provide examples of each type of quality care cut. Do you agree or disagree that these quality care cuts are necessary? If yes, then what are the consequences if these cuts are not taken?

9. Do you think that assistants who provide care to seniors without speaking or with behaving with indifference and apathy are psychologically abusive? Some studies demonstrate that these behaviors happen only on an occasional basis. How frequently, if at all, should an administrator tolerate this behavior from an assistant? Provide suggestions to prevent this type of behavior from assistants.

10. Most frontline staff members complete their work in spite of their low wages. What seems to motivate these staff to come to work and do a good job? How can administrators ensure that these motivating factors are in the work environment on a daily basis?

11. Several areas of dissatisfaction were identified by assistants including low wages, and supervisor and manager problems. What evidence would you need as an administrator that these areas had improved for your assistants?

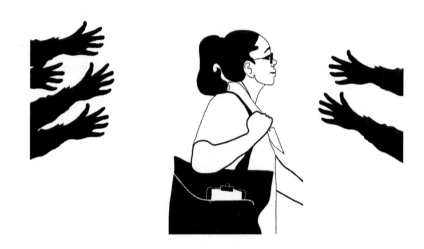

"The seniors have so many needs. I've never done enough for each one."

CHAPTER 4

VOICES OF NURSES

> The well educated nurse is at the
> heart of elder health care and
> provides an indispensable level
> of competence for which there is
> no substitute.[1]

Although nurses are the smallest segment of the long-term care staff, they have a significant impact on seniors and on those with whom they work. Seminal studies have found that nursing homes with high nurse-to-senior ratios have half as many seniors with bed sores and incontinence as those with low nurse-to-senior ratios. Moreover, nursing homes with low nurse-to-senior ratios incur more state violations and experience higher staff turnover.[2, 3, 4]

Two types of nurses are employed by long-term care organizations: registered nurses (RNs) and licensed practical nurses (LPNs). Licensed practical nurses have graduated from approved practical nursing programs (which range from eight months to two years in length) and have successfully passed a state-level standardized examination. They are considered a vital part of health care teams and generally conduct a large share of direct patient care.[5] Licensed practical nurses make up the majority of nurses in nursing homes and assisted-living facilities but the smallest segment of the home care industry, representing about 20% of home health care employees and only about 6% of workers in Medicare certified agencies.[6] In whichever setting they work, they are paid much more than frontline assistants but considerably less than RNs.

Registered nurses have a variety of educational backgrounds: they have successfully completed one of the following: a two-year college program, a four-year college or university program, or a hospital-based, college-enhanced program. All registered nurses must pass a national-level examination and abide by state nurse practice acts and guidelines. Registered nurses generally have the ultimate responsibility for conducting clinical procedures prescribed by physicians. Additionally, they are responsible for seeing that quality standards are enforced among those workers in their charge and that compliance with state and local regulations is assured. Often LPNs act as charge nurses over assistants, but the registered nurse (RN) conducts the annual evaluations and monitors seniors' clinical statuses. Medicare and Medicaid have strict guidelines for RN oversight in home care services and nursing home care, with minimum requirements set per every 100 seniors.

Financial Management

Financial management tasks include analyzing financial statements and budgets along with assets and revenue management. Specific tasks include developing and evaluating the organization's budget, monitoring financial obligations, and approving and monitoring vendor contracts and department budgets. The majority of home care and nursing home executives feel that maximizing reimbursements and optimizing overall financial performance were some of their top priorities, and they spent a large proportion of their time dealing with financial matters.[9] Directors of nursing, however, do not manage organizational or departmental finances as much as they would like. Most directors felt this was due to the demands of other, more pressing, matters; although some directors of nursing felt barred from access to financial information by their administrators.[10]

This chapter is based on studies of nurses in long-term care settings. These studies vary by intent from identifying job satisfaction areas and general nursing tasks to recording and analyzing nurses' descriptions of their work life challenges. The majority of studies are surveys with Likert rating scales; however, several qualitative studies including focus groups, open-ended interviews, and systematic observations, are included. All studies focused on listening to nurses' voices and considering their actions in long-term care organizations. Assisted-living facilities are the newest area in which long-term care nurses work (nearly 70% of these facilities hire nurses), and systematic studies of these nurses were not found. Nevertheless, a few articles interviewing assisted-living nurses have been published, and quotes from these sources are included throughout this chapter.

This chapter provides descriptions of a typical day by nursing home, assisted-living, and home care nurses. It then continues with more details of the daily functions that these nurses regularly perform in long-term care settings. Some activities such as teaching are performed more frequently by home care nurses, while other activities such as supervising are performed more frequently by assisted-living and nursing home nurses. The chapter continues by reporting nurses' satisfactions and reasons for working in long-term care organizations. Last, nurses' challenges and reasons for burnout are examined. Additionally, nurses' actions as they interact with clients are observed, and the joys of their jobs and particularly proud moments are heard.

Typical Days

Nurses in three long-term care settings—nursing homes, assisted-living facilities and home care agencies—were asked what their typical days were like. Many nurses said that every day was different, but then they were asked to think about a recent day and just recount the day's activities. One discouraged nursing home nurse described her day as never ending responsibilities with daily emotional stress as a consequence of being confronted with deaths, and the failing health and loneliness of residents.[7] She then described her day as "a constant interaction between job responsibilities, needs of the seniors, staff shortages, limited resources and lack of time."[8] A more tangible description of a typical day given by a nurse is: "Passing meds to 35—40 people, taking care of all the treatments, doctors' orders, charting, overseeing all the nurse's aides, and dealing with people that are in a crisis situation." [9]

Typical days in assisted-living facilities seem less stressful as the seniors do not have as many health problems; however, the nurse does not have as much support staff. As one nurse said,

> Working in assisted-living is a holistic approach to nursing. We are making sure that seniors are socially well adjusted, and that their psychosocial and physical needs are met. The dynamics of interacting with the seniors and the ability that the nurse has to enhance the quality of life for that senior are just fabulous. The focus on senior independence and seniors' dictation of their care plan are to some degree unique to assisted-living. [10]

In most assisted-living facilities, the training and supervision of UAPs (unlicensed assistive personnel) is a daily responsibility of the nurse, along with monitoring seniors' health status, being a family liaison, and making health service appointments.[11]

Home care nurses have scheduling flexibility but, when listening to descriptions of their typical days, they seem to perform the same duties within each work day. One home care nurse described her day as follows:

> My day usually starts at 7 on the telephone [connecting by computer to get fresh orders and then calling to schedule appointments]...I usually see my first patient between 7:30 and 8. I go in and take temperature and blood pressure and talk to them. A lot of times the people we see are homebound and the only people they see in the day are us. . . .I dress the wound, and that's about 45 minutes, and I finish charting and go on to the next one. I chart between visits and generally am done by 2. I come into the office and export my stuff. Paper work is never ending. I'm done between 3 & 4, usually. [12]

Each home care agency has different work arrangements. Some agencies have nurses who do all the first visits ("admissions"), and some spread the admissions evenly among all their home care nurses. Another home care nurse described her day as, "Typically I see 6 or 7 people in a day and I travel around and visit them in their homes. Sometimes I have admissions to home care and those take longer. More of our time is spent doing paperwork than care. We draw blood, do dressing changes, and help [clients] with tube feedings if they have those."[13] Paperwork refers to the insurance forms (primarily Medicare) the nurses need to complete to get fully reimbursed. Dependent on the home care agency, nurses may complete this "paperwork" either with paper and pen or with agency supplied computers. A job analysis of home care nurses working in different agencies found that home care nurses average four to five patient visits per day, with the first visit after a hospitalization taking almost twice as long as other visits (this is the "admissions visit"). Interestingly, when average times for salaried nurses and nurses paid per visit were compared, the salaried nurses were more efficient, spending less time charting.[14]

Daily Functions

Generally, nurses have very little awareness of the daily functions of other nurses working in healthcare settings different from their own. In one study, home care nurses admitted that their clients often needed other kinds of care, but they just did not know how to coordinate or integrate care beyond their own settings.[15] In another study, nurses who shared clients from one setting to another (i.e., hospital to home care) met to discuss their mutual clients and were often surprised at each others' multiple duties and responsibilities.[16] In focus groups of home care and hospital nurses, hospital nurses identified misconceptions regarding their clients' available support and abilities to function in their own homes. After these group discussions, hospital nurses were determined to work on improving the education and written directions they gave senior clients upon discharge. They also planned on discussing with their senior client a more realistic picture of what needed to be done in their homes and the limits of what home health nurses could do. Basically, the hospital nurses recognized that both they and their senior clients had inflated expectations of the actual amount of time, on average, that home care nurses would spend providing care. Many thought nurses would perform clinical tasks, rather than teaching seniors or their family members to care for themselves.[17] This lack of effective communication is found between nursing home nurses and hospital nurses as well. Generally, nurses agree that more effective communication among all long-term care nurses is needed so they can be more sensitive to each other and enhance care as well.

Four nursing activities have been identified as common among long-term care nurses; they are direct care, caring and connecting, teaching, and supervising and managing. These four roles encompass the essential core activities of long-term care nurses. The most common activity is "direct care" and requires hands-on client care (often using clinical skills.)[18] Caring and connecting is the psychosocial care given by nurses, often at the same time as direct care is given. The teaching activity refers to both instructing clients how to care for themselves as well as teaching nursing assistants. Supervising and managing refers to coordinating nursing assistants as well as other tasks required to keep the overall organization working at its best. In addition to these basic roles, managers of nurses have identified characteristics of outstanding nurses—those things that separate a nurse giving exceptional care from an average nurse. These characteristics are: giving person-centered care, being gerontological clinical experts, and supporting team-builders.[19] Each of these characteristics was found as extra touches that exceptional nurses brought to their daily activities.

Nurses in different long-term care settings distribute their time among the essential daily activities very differently, and even within the same setting, nurses often differ significantly in the percentage of time they devote to various tasks. Job analysis studies of nurses reveal the amount of time they spend doing specific tasks. One study of nearly 3,000 nurses working in nursing homes found that nurses spend the greatest proportion of their days, about 44%, in direct client care. Indirect activities, such as staff supervision, comprise about 30% of a nurse's day, and administrative duties account for the remaining 26%.[20] Three home care studies in which nurses kept daily logs found that nurses spend high proportions of their time in indirect care. The first study, conducted in 1988, found that direct care activities consumed about 29% of a home care nurse's day. The remaining indirect care work was divided among charting, correspondence for client care, recertification-related paperwork, travel, and supervision of home care assistants.[21] Another job analysis of 400 home care nurses conducted five years later found a higher average time spent in giving direct care to seniors. This study found that 62% of nurses' time was spent on direct patient care, 15% on administrative activities, and 14% on consulting.[22] A third study of home care nurses found that they took an average of 112 minutes to complete all activities related to one patient visit. Forty-seven percent of this time was spent on direct patient care, and the rest was spent on travel, charting, and professional communication or referrals.[23]

Direct Care

Direct care activities include observable care provided to clients such as distributing medications, changing dressings or colostomies, checking blood glucose levels, and performing physical assessments. Direct care also includes invisible care which directly impacts seniors' health, such as calling a physician regarding a changed vital sign, developing care plans, monitoring seniors' health goals and interventions, conducting care conferences regarding the seniors' progress, or checking clients' insurance coverage.[24]

Nurses in all long-term care settings provide direct care. In assisted-living facilities, few assessments involve life-saving decisions, but nurses are often the only medical professional on site. These nurses often impact seniors' health by noticing the early signs of dehydration or symptoms of respiratory infection. In emergencies, they call 911 or the family. If the family does not respond, it is up to the nurse to stay on the problem and get the desired outcome.[25] Over ninety percent of assisted-living facility nurses are on call after hours, just to perform direct care when needed. [26]

Most direct care activities are done in different proportions as long-term care settings differ by clients' needs. Focus groups found some differences between nursing home nurses and hospital nurses. Nurses in acute care had more standardized care plans and treatment interventions. As one nurse said, "We have standardized care plans, and you just highlight the parts that fit your patients." [27] Nursing home nurses described their direct care routines differently, considering individualization and creativity more important. One nursing home nurse said that direct care required knowledge of the seniors, their personal history and previous responses to nursing and medical management.[28]

Caring & Connecting

Nurses in all long-term care settings make significant contributions to seniors within the psychological domain. Clients benefit physically and emotionally from nurses' support and connectedness. Caring skills are developed from experience and continuing relationships with clients. Long-term care nurses come to know their clients over time and in multiple dimensions, using this knowledge in caring for them.[29]

Several home care nurses mentioned that to connect meaningfully with these individual's clients, they have to suspend their own values and really listen to these clients. The nurses emphasized that in entering homes where the values or lifestyles were different from their own that the key to success was accepting everyone no matter how ideas and priorities differed. Home care nurses emphasized that to gain entrance and serve well they needed to establish trust and rapport quickly. These nurses often cited their greatest strength as interpersonal skills.[30]

A good example of a home care nurse really listening to and supporting her client follows. While providing care, the nurse heard her client make an offhand remark about having no food, but nothing further was said about it. As the nurse left the home, she checked in the refrigerator and several cabinets. She went right back upstairs, explained what she had done and why, and then together, the nurse and client worked on the problem.[31]

Two studies which recorded senior-staff interactions in nursing homes and independent-living facilities found that nurses' communication styles were generally positive and caring. Most nurses were uplifting while they were in seniors' rooms, making many autonomy-valuing statements and encouraging seniors to be as independent as possible.[32, 33] Both studies found that nurses talked much more with the seniors than assistants did. Many times nurses tried to get conversations going with seniors, seeking their opinions and having them decide on daily care routines.

In some conversations about nursing care, some nurses implied "caring" as a sort of client advocacy. Many researchers were surprised by the intensity of the nurses' indignation as they discussed the potential effects of a label such as "confused" and the treatment of older adults as objects. When talking about confusion, one nurse commented about the mental status test:

> What is the date, anyway? To so many of my patients that is an unfair question. If they know the season after they have been on the unit for weeks, then I check them as correct for orientation to time. . . .When they are sick, they don't care about the date. I understand that.[34]

In summary, "caring and connecting" seems to be an essential part of the job for all long-term care nurses. This daily task takes a variety of forms, dependent on the seniors as well as the nurses. Above all, caring and connecting means providing personal recognition to seniors and encouraging their autonomy and independence.

Teaching

Teaching is often thought of as only instructing clients and family members in how to complete clinical procedures; however long-term care nurses identify teaching as much more than this. Long-term care nurses identified teaching as both instructions and advocacy for their clients and as something necessary for other healthcare professionals with whom they worked. One nursing home nurse said, "I think nursing's greatest impact is in senior advocacy." Typically, the nurse goes to bat for the patient saying, "This med routine is not working; let's come up with something new."[35] Then she helps the client develop her questions for the physician. Many seniors' insurance is now handled by managed care organizations and they face the challenges of the restrictive conditions imposed. Often nurses were found advocating for their seniors and seeking coverage for the care they need. Home care nurses, too, felt that they must advocate for their clients. Often they found referral sources and other help for their elderly clients.

Monitoring and training staff was also recognized as a daily teaching activity of nurses. Both nursing home and assisted-living facility nurses often mentioned that they felt especially responsible to monitor unlicensed staff members who were passing medications in their facilities. Home care nurses are responsible for monitoring home care assistants' notes and often are on-call to these assistants whenever they have questions regarding their clients. Often home care nurses are responsible for providing short in-services to home care assistants regarding general client care tasks.[36]

Many nurses found teaching their clients very satisfying. Several home care nurses told stories about patients who were initially difficult to work with, but who responded positively to their efforts. One example was a man discharged from the hospital with a new colostomy. He was very angry and often rude to the nurse, complaining that she refused to do his care while she insisted her job was to teach him to care for the colostomy, himself. He was re-hospitalized, but when he was again discharged, he requested the same nurse and he learned to care for the colostomy.[37]

With current reimbursement home care nurses are expected to provide more teaching so clients can quickly learn to care for themselves. This can be especially challenging in home care, as the nurses noted that the home can be more distracting with personal phone calls, family visits, and home appliances running. They do set limits with their clients and have identified teaching methods that work especially well. These are: 1) emphasizing serious consequences and high chances of illness recurrence as an incentive to learn, 2) identifying major problem areas and then tackling one problem at a time, and 3) capitalizing on learner frustration, convincing clients that positive benefits can result from particular behaviors.[38]

Supervising and Managing

Supervision is a significant activity nurses in long-term care organizations must perform daily. Supervision is usually of nursing assistants for nursing home nurses, home care aides for home care nurses, and unlicensed assistants for assisted-living nurses. In organizations with licensed practical nurses, registered nurses were expected to supervise these nurses, as well. Nurses in all long-term care organizations consistently identified supervision as an activity they did not enjoy; in addition, they did not often feel qualified to do it. They recognized that someone needed to supervise the direct care staff, but found this task particularly distasteful and thankless.

Nurse managers interviewed about the supervision skills of their registered nurses were found to be generally unhappy. They praised many of their nurses for their senior focus and assessment skills, but noted that their nurses consistently had difficulty performing necessary supervision of LPNs and nursing assistants. Nurses often needed reminders to delegate tasks to nursing assistants and to supervise nursing assistant performance more carefully. The managers noted that nurses often just could not supervise the more difficult nursing assistants. Furthermore, conducting performance evaluations, giving constructive criticism, and making suggestions for improvement were tremendous challenges. Interestingly, these same nurse managers noted their organizations offered no in-house coursework or professional development workshops in supervision or other management areas.[39]

Another study examined nurses' involvement in managerial decisions as perceived by administrators of nursing homes. Nurses were primarily involved in organizational policies regarding senior care as opposed to strategic operations or marketing. Nurses' primary method of managerial involvement was identifying care issues, and it was recognized that the nurses seldom were involved in managerial problem solving on these issues. If they were involved, it was often through informal conversations with administrators.[40] In nursing homes that had greater nurses' involvement in managerial decisions, the clients were found to have had better health and functioning. Specifically, after six months of nurses more directly participating in managerial decisions, seniors experienced less dehydration and fewer decubitus ulcers, urinary tract infections, fractures, and contractures.[41]

Clearly, long-term care nurses have a role that extends beyond direct clinical care, caring, and teaching activities. Nurses seem to recognize the necessity of supervising and that they are not performing it most effectively. Nevertheless, many may not realize the significant clinical impact improved supervision and direct managerial participation can have on the seniors under their care.

Values and Satisfactions

The values a person brings to a job can be enabled and fostered by the right leadership and management, or obstructed by incompatible leadership and management. One of the essential tasks of an effective administrator is to listen to and consider the values and levels of professional satisfaction of their staff. Core values and satisfactions can easily be concealed by the multiple demands of clients and the rush of daily duties. On the other hand, neglecting nurses' core values can lead to negative work attitudes, burnout, and high turnover.

In reviewing studies of long-term care nurses, the nurses repeatedly mentioned three significant areas of satisfaction.[42] First, the ability to provide care and comfort to individuals was sincerely valued. Many nurses felt they were "making a difference" in someone's life, and it felt intrinsically good to them. Second, nurses valued the opportunity to care for a whole person—physically, socially, and psychologically. Many times nurses mentioned how great it was to really know their patients and how they valued the time they spent with them. They felt that the care they provided was much more than just ministering to physical health needs. Theses two values—comforting and making a difference, and relating to a whole person—were by far the most frequently cherished aspects of long-term care nurses' jobs. A third value recognized by home care nurses was professional autonomy and growth.[43] Nurses in nursing homes and assisted-living facilities occasionally mentioned professional growth, but home care nurses nearly always identified this area as very satisfying. One home care nurse stated, "I've nursed for 15 years, but I was never really a nurse until I started doing home health nursing."[44]

Giving Comfort and Making a Difference

Only one study asked long-term care nurses about their values directly. This study dealt with nurses who worked with seniors suffering from various stages of dementia.[45] The researchers gave nurses cards which listed facility character-istics and personal characteristics. For each set of cards, the nurse was asked to rank them by importance to her or him. The facility characteristics nurses valued as most important for providing quality care were teamwork, administrative support, staff attitudes, and knowledge. Administrative support was defined as giving staff enough time to give good care, while "staff attitudes" was defined as willingness to spend time with seniors, giving more than just physical care. The top personal values were genuinely liking individuals with dementia, being flexible, being kind and calm, and having a positive attitude.[46] Clearly, these values, whether labeled as facility or personal characteristics, are very client centered and focus on nurses caring for their clients.

Caring values were also found in a study in which nurses were asked to talk about their professional satisfactions. Researchers asked nurses, "Tell us about a day when you returned home and thought, 'Today was a good day.'"[47] Embar-rassed looks were exchanged until one nurse said, "I don't think that has ever happened to me—a whole day."[48] It became clear that the nurses did not feel they could answer this question, so the research question was changed to, "Tell us about rewarding moments."[49] In response to this modified request, nurses shared many memorable stories about their experiences with clients.

One home care nurse described a particularly proud experience she had with one elderly client.[50] This nurse had a senior who kept losing weight, and she discovered the senior wasn't eating because she was afraid of choking as her dentures were too big. The senior had Medicaid insurance, which no dentist in the area accepted. After many calls, the nurse found a dentist accepting Medi-caid and assisted the senior in finding transportation to the dentist to get new dentures. The senior began eating again. "The best part is assisting clients to stay in their own homes and having them succeed in society."[51]

During interviews, nurses often compared their days in hospitals with their current long-term care positions. In one interview, a nursing home nurse said, "In the hospital, your basic agenda is life saving. In this facility [a nursing home], your basic thing is comfort and quality of care."[52] A home care nurse remarked, "The most exciting aspects of home health care nurses' work are the ability to make a difference in patients' lives, to be an important part of the health care team and achieve improved patient outcomes."[53]

In another study, nurses answered the question, "What's the best thing about working here?"[54] The majority of nurses in all long-term care organiza-tions said that the best part of their jobs was caring for their patients and doing worthwhile work. One nursing home nurse said, "I like the feeling that you're doing something for the senior and making life just a little easier for them beings they have to be here."[55]

Caring for the Whole Person

Many times in conversations, nurses mentioned that a particularly reward-ing aspect of long-term care is really getting to know patients and their families. Many nurses in nursing homes and assisted-living facilities emphasized how close they felt to their clients because they had known them and their families for so long. One nursing home nurse said, "I guess why I have chosen to stay in this type of setting [nursing home] is I enjoy seeing the patients for a lot longer stay than in the hospital. It's nice to get to know the patients and their fami-lies."[56]

Home care nurses gave many related examples in a study in which they were asked to describe times they felt really proud of their work.[57] They re-ported that their relationships with seniors in their homes yielded many such moments. They often got to develop trusting relationships with their patients, relationships that were just not possible in hospitals. They knew both personal information about and feelings of their patients, their family members, and their challenges. One nurse reported making a home visit and finding her patient's husband in more need than the patient. The nurse was able to get help for him, which, in turn, calmed her patient.[58]

Home care nurses said that the ability to give their complete attention to just one patient in the comfort of his or her own home was the best part of their jobs. These things gave them the opportunity to really relate to patients and their cir-cumstances. These nurses often emphasized this one-to-one aspect of their work. One nurse stated, "The best is the ability to spend time with the patients. It is being a primary care nurse and managing the care. You can provide the best care possible in their environment."[59] Some home care nurses expressed their satis-faction at having the time to meet the many aspects of patients' needs. One nurse said,

> I feel like I'm more fulfilled because when I'm sitting down with a patient, I don't have to run to another room because somebody needs pain medication or somebody needs to be suctioned or whatever. I feel like I can sit with this patient and focus on him and we're not go-ing to be interrupted unless it's by another family member.[60]

One final tribute to the joy of such relationships was made by a nurse with almost 30 years' experience in skilled-nursing facilities. "Seniors and families have always given me more than I feel I gave them in return. I've learned from them—learned how to cope in difficult times—learned what's important in life and how to look at things and not have regrets." [61]

Professional Autonomy and Growth

In addition to caring for their patients, home care nurses acknowledge an-other aspect of their jobs which they consider significant—professional autonomy and consistent growth. Several studies found that the majority of home care nurses report the most satisfying areas of their work as the close client relationships and sense of making a difference; however, professional autonomy and practice of their work was also valued and identified as the top satisfier for many home care nurses. As one nurse put it, "The best thing is that I'm in control of what I do."[62]

In a focus group, one nurse said that home health was the last positive place to practice nursing.[63] In general home care nurses reported growth in their clinical skills, in communicating with other health care providers, in assertiveness, and in self-direction. Another nurse concurred, "I've never had a job where you could grow so much… It has made me grow as a person and professionally more than any other job in nursing would have. In home care you need to be responsible…"[64]

In discussions among home care nurses, professional autonomy was described as walking a fine line in connecting with, tending to, and releasing their clients. The nurses said that they had to take a broad view of everything that affected their clients and know when they needed to "finish." This meant educating the clients, preparing them to be independent, and then letting them go.[65]

Job Satisfaction

Administrators are generally interested in nurses' job satisfaction for two reasons: (a) they do not want their nurses seeking jobs elsewhere and (b) happy, satisfied nurses provide better care to clients, especially needy, elderly persons. Many studies have validated these reasons.

RN turnover rates in nursing homes range from 55 to 65 %.[66] Several studies have found that nurses with higher satisfaction ratings in specific job areas intend to stay longer.[67] Specifically, nurses who intend to stay in their current positions have higher satisfaction with their professional status, job autonomy, interactions with other nurses, and salaries. Also, these long-term care nurses believe their supervisors are concerned about them and their careers.[68]

Older clients in nursing homes, as well as those receiving home care services, rate their satisfaction and sense of caring from the nursing staff higher when their nurses are more satisfied.[69] These findings are particularly significant as they validate that seniors can see a difference in their personal care and sense of caring, just by the professional job satisfaction of their nurses.

Are long-term care nurses generally satisfied, and in what areas do they have the most and least satisfaction? Home care and nursing home nurses report slightly higher rates of satisfaction than do hospital nurses. Then again, neither group of nurses are very satisfied; even home care nurses' highest ratings are in the range of "neutral satisfaction."[70,71, 72] Congruent with their identified values, home care nurses experience more satisfaction with job involvement, the opportunity to determine methods and procedures, and the opportunity to share in goal-setting. They also had more intrinsic satisfaction, which was composed of their opportunity to participate in important and worthwhile activities.[73] Nursing home nurses' highest satisfaction was in patient care and relationships with coworkers. Their lowest satisfaction was with their work load and supervisors.[74]

Dissatisfactions and Professional Challenges

Several researchers have noted that long-term care nurses were much more inclined to speak about their satisfaction than about their areas of discontent. However, when pushed, nurses did identify areas of dissatisfaction. Additionally, during interviews, nurses almost inadvertently mentioned areas of their jobs they were unhappy with in the course of describing their activities. Internal conflict within their organizations or between their own values and demanded activities often resulted in a variety of negative attitudes and job dissatisfaction, which was not explicitly recognized until interviewers questioned the nurses directly and pulled this information out.

Four areas of dissatisfaction were consistently found among long-term care nurses: relationships with supervisors and administrators, work overload, documentation demands, and low salaries. Nurses in both home care and nursing homes gave examples of their unhappiness in each of these areas. One significant job area, professional respect, was perceived oppositely by nurses in nursing homes versus home care nurses. This seems to be a powerful component of job satisfaction; each perspective is examined in a later section in this chapter.

Supervisors and Administrators

Negative feelings toward supervisors were one of nurses' most common complaints. In fact, managerial inadequacy and supervisor deficiencies are the primary complaints from long-term care nurses in all settings. On a five-point scale, supervisors were rated dissatisfactory or very dissatisfactory, both in home care agencies and in nursing homes.[75, 76] Lack of recognition or any praise at all for nurses' dedication to their clients and their willingness to help during short-handed shifts were often mentioned as a dispiriting aspect of their jobs.

These ratings have important implications. Studies in both home care agencies and nursing homes found that negative feelings towards supervisors are the primary component of the workplace driving nurses to leave their jobs. Likewise, studies found that when nurses believe that their supervisors are interested in them as people and professionals, they have stronger commitments to stay with their employers.[77, 78] In a similar vein, respect for supervisors is very important. One study found that when nurses felt that their supervisors were respected within the community and by other long-term care organizations, they felt much more committed to their work and their futures in the nursing home.[79]

With recognition of dissatisfaction in this area, nurses were asked what type of supervision they would like. Nurses mentioned supportive leadership, which is friendly and approachable. They wanted their supervisors to have a clear understanding of their jobs and their challenges, and to look out for the needs of both the clients and staff. Most nurses felt they did not need much direction, just support and respect for their opinions and hard work.[80] The feeling of having someone they can trust and turn to when things got tough was thoroughly appreciated.

Workload Overload

During interviews, most home care and nursing home nurses mentioned having too much to do for their clients. Many nurses mentioned they wished they had more time to listen and visit, to know seniors, and be more patient. Sometimes these comments were voiced as complaints, and at other times, they were framed as just the reality of the job. In describing their days, several nursing home nurses stated that their (heavy) workload was not due to poor staffing as they had the "state-required ratio."[81] One nurse claimed, "We have the minimum amount of staff that we need to have for the state, but it still doesn't seem to go far enough."[82] Another nurse said, "There are a lot of people that we are in charge of during the day. . . It's not that we're short staffed, but it's just impossible to get everything done."[83]

These comments are surprising in consideration of the small amount of time nurses have to devote to each senior each day. Although there is much variance within and among nursing homes, current RN-to-senior ratios in nursing homes average 1 nurse per 49 seniors compared to a ratio of 1 RN per every 4 patients in a hospital. Another survey reported an overall average of 6.3 RNs per 100 beds, which, when converted to hours, yielded an average nurse's time per senior per day of 21 minutes. In 1985, the median amount of RN time per senior per day in American nursing homes was 12 minutes or less and nearly 40% reported 6 minutes or less of RN time per senior per day.[84] It is refreshing to see that time has improved this situation. Wide variations in staffing patterns have been found across metropolitan areas of the U.S. and among Medicaid-only nursing homes versus those with more diversified funding sources.[85, 86]

Home health care nurses mentioned workload frustration as well. Most frequently nurses complained about the highly acute needs of their clients and the number of clients they were expected to see each day; however, new areas of concern, such as learning insurance requirements and new regulation forms, were also mentioned. Sometimes the problem was labeled "time management"; yet, when the nurses started listing all they had to do in eight hours—regular visits, new admissions, documentation, driving, phone arrangements, and staff meetings—it was clear there was work overload.[87] In one home care study nurses were asked what changes were needed in their jobs. While a narrow set of desired changes could not be developed, over 50% of the nurses complained about workload issues. They made comments about their expected productivity goals, lack of control of schedules, and multiple tasks required, from learning new technology and regulations to supervising assistants and attending required staff meetings.[88]

The rising level of seriousness in clients' health problems was a concern for many home care nurses. Nearly all had stories of their experiences with patients discharged early with highly acute needs. Nurses felt the need to provide not only good clinical care, but also emotional support. As one said, "The patients are already stressed from the hospitalization, but then are doubly stressed when they get home and suddenly realize they have a bag, they have a line, and this needle in their arm."[89] Some nurses reported that early discharges of aging clients threw families into crisis, as often every family member was working, leaving no caregiver in the home. This added problems associated with angry family members and nurses trying to determine the safety of elders left alone. Nurses also reported that mental health diagnoses have increased and fewer patients are admitted for surgery, which left home care nurses to do post-operative assessments following out-patient surgeries.[90]

Another concern of home care nurses was the limitations in the number of visits allowed that are often imposed by insurance companies and changing Medicare guidelines. Nurses felt very responsible for seeing that their clients were safe and healing well, yet they were pressured to provide very few visits. One nurse spoke about a man discharged early, with surgical staples still in place after a coronary bypass. He was allowed two visits: an initial assessment, and another visit to remove the staples. She said she had wanted to visit after she took out the staples just to inspect the incision, ensure he could shower, and was not experiencing chest pain. The insurance company denied her request.[91]

Dissatisfaction with workloads is similar for nursing home nurses, but is not identified on survey scales as frequently. In one nursing home study, a nurse said, "When you start in the morning with fewer than three nurses, then you think oh, today's going to be busy, and I'll have to work very hard. But no matter how much I help the seniors, it doesn't do them any good...You don't have time to spend half an hour helping (seniors), because there are so many others waiting for you to come and help them. Every day is a race against the clock."[92]

Documentation Requirements

Necessary documentation in long-term care has grown tremendously with the prospective payment systems imposed by Medicare cost control and quality monitoring programs. The regulations require detailed assessments of every client multiple times throughout the year. These documents vary from 10 to 40 pages per client. For nursing homes, these regulations and documents (DRG or Diagnosis Related Groups and MDS or Minimum Data Set regulations) have been in place since the early 1990s, while home care agencies started their system (OASIS or Outcomes and Assessment Information Set regulations) around 2000. Each year, changes are made to the systems, and data reports to organizations are improved. Still, nurses were often heard talking about their frustrations with the systems' inflexibility and inadequacy to meet patient needs.

Nursing home nurses appear less frustrated than home care nurses, and some even acknowledge these documents' value. Nurses from both settings, however, seem to enjoy outwitting regulations to benefit clients. One nursing home study reported that most nurses seemed to comply with regulatory restrictions. Regulations concerning the financing of the nursing homes seem respected as important in modifying patient care—in determining where, for what causes, and for how long patients and seniors could reside in the nursing home. However, during one of the taped weekly discharge planning meetings, a therapist asked that the tape be turned off. He then told the researcher of preventing patients from walking 100 feet if that would necessitate termination of the patient's physical therapy reimbursement while other needs remained to be met.[93] In a different study, a home care nurse related a similar story of outwitting the

system in making arrangements for a woman with cancer to go home for terminal care. This patient had no family and had been receiving services from a program for abused women. The nurse arranged for another abused woman to move
into the patient's home and serve as her caregiver. She commented, "I felt real
good when we got her home. She wanted to go home, and it's hard to take some-
body home who has no money and no family."[94, 95]

Home care nurses find regulations and required documentation much more
overwhelming than do nursing home nurses. Their biggest complaints center
around the extraordinary volume of paperwork required for each home visit.
Some claimed that it interfered with their client care, delaying the provision of
clinical care and support. One study compared nurses in agencies which provided computers for charting with nurses in agencies which still used paper-
based charting, but both complained vehemently about documentation demands.[96] One home care nurse said, "The worst [aspect of work] is the paperwork. It's more than I've done in other areas of nursing. There are so many
guidelines and how they apply. My documentation has to be superb to make sure
we get maximum reimbursement."[97] Another home care nurse commented,
"OASIS is 100% paperwork and has nothing to do with the patients. Why can't
they come up with 10 questions instead of 17 pages....It's killing us. I'm to the
point that I don't care if I do my job or not. I love the patients, but the stress
level around here is enormous."[98]

Another study of home care nurses reported that some nurses were feeling
great stress and pressure from the underlying implications of documentation
regulations. Some nurses stated they resented the sense of being scrutinized and
having to document every little thing. Yet other nurses in this same study felt the
burden of financial responsibility to their employing agencies: "You are holding
the bag, being responsible to the patient, to the family, to the community and
just a little thing will get past you...something you didn't document...and the
agency will lose money because you let something slip by."[99]

On a contrary note, an interview with one nurse who had worked in nursing
homes for 30 years did not find the regulatory documentation entirely negative:
"Although a lot more is required of nurses now, I feel that each regulation has
improved senior care....I feel that it is a comprehensive, holistic document that
really looks at every detail pertinent to the senior—if it's done right." This nurse
admitted that regulations are difficult to follow and intimidating, but said that
without them, nursing homes could become lax.[100]

Salary Dissatisfaction

Several studies have found that both home care and nursing home nurses
are dissatisfied with their salaries.[101] Salaries have long been lower in nursing
homes than in acute care settings. This may be because nursing home reimbursements are primarily dependent on state and federal funding. In the 1990s,
nursing home RN salaries were about 15% lower than salaries for hospital
RNs.[102] Recent national surveys revealed that pay hikes have occurred for nursing home nurses, but a registered nurse in a nursing home still averages less pay
than a hospital nurse. However, the salary distribution was just the opposite for

LPNs. These nurses actually have slightly higher average salaries in assisted-living facilities and nursing homes than they do in hospitals.[103]

Professional Respect, Satisfaction, and Dissatisfaction

One study of nurses in four nursing homes and all the physicians who had three or more seniors in those homes found significant disrespect for nurses.[104] MDs gave significantly low ratings for nurses being able to distinguish urgent from non-urgent problems and in being able to identify problems in a timely manner. Furthermore, they felt nurses did not know how to assess patients before they called them or to explain perceived problems clearly and concisely. They felt many calls were trivial or unnecessary. Nurses, not surprisingly, felt physicians were not pleasant during their phone calls and did not respect or value their professional opinions. Nurses reported that physicians were frequently difficult to reach, often did not return phone calls promptly, and were sometimes irritated by calls they perceived as insignificant. Physicians reported their decision-making process was compromised by nurses' poor assessment and inadequate communication of changes in a senior's condition. This led them to order hospitalization prior to any real identified need.

Just the opposite is found in terms of professional respect for home care nurses. These nurses reported collegial relationships with many physicians. Frequently, physicians said, "Do whatever you think is best. I'll sign the orders."[105] In addition to respect from physicians, some nurses felt respect from administration. In one instance, a health maintenance organization (HMO) gave a nurse freedom to provide any services she thought necessary to keep a chronic obstructive lung disease patient out of the hospital for the winter. (The nurse was creative and successful in preventing further hospitalization.)[106] Another study of North Dakota home care nurses found that professional status was their highest area of job satisfaction.[107]

Burnout

Burned out professionals are defined as having "depleted or exhausted their emotional and physical energies in dealing with the stressors of the work environment."[108] Some studies have found that a higher percentage of nursing home nurses than hospital nurses suffer from moderate burnout through emotional exhaustion and depersonalization.[109]

The impact of burned out nurses on clients is serious. Studies both in United States and Swedish nursing homes have found that nurses scoring high in burnout had less empathy, attitudes less positive towards the elderly, and a greater tendency to depersonalize their clients.[110, 111] Another study found that nurses avoided seniors to cope with burnout. They would regularly avoid talking with the seniors, and interacting in any situations and activities which demanded empathy.[112] Nurses who used this depersonalization strategy made it very clear that they were either too busy doing something or having a break in order to prevent seniors from asking for something. These nurses avoided talking about difficult or emotional subjects with patients, participating in only those conversations which did not present a threat. One nurse said,

> There is always something practical that needs doing, so to speak.
> You have the idea that you always have to tidy up the ward, for ex-
> ample. I have to do something, to start doing something like cutting
> nails, watering flowers or stocking up the cupboards.[113]

One extensive study of nurses examined job satisfaction and burnout in terms of how long nurses have been at their jobs.[114] The researchers found different influences on nurses' satisfaction areas at different times. Nurses who had worked three to six years were the most likely to be burned out. They may have been thinking, "Is this all there is?" and wondering about the significance of their work and needing to be shown that their work is important. Nurses who had worked six months to one year were at the highest turnover intention stage and were the most dissatisfied. Raw recruits and nurses with fewer than six months of work needed feedback to make sure they were doing their jobs well. Nurses who had worked six months to one year were the only group for whom payoff for good work was important; also important were co-workers' feedback and perceived job autonomy. Nurses who had worked one to three years had the lowest dissatisfaction related to turnover intent. Some nursing homes have used support groups to help staff handle stress or have combined in-service education with support teams for nurses suffering burnout. Other approaches nursing homes have used are changing staffing patterns, shifting workloads, and negotiating staff assignments.[115]

Conclusion

Long-term care offers nurses opportunities unavailable in acute care settings. Getting to know patients as people is just not possible in an environment of prospective payments and continually compressed hospital stays. Likewise, the opportunity for home care nurses to be in control, "using all the knowledge and skills we were taught in school" is a unique benefit not available in acute care settings with stressed physicians pressured by compliance monitoring. Yet, these intrinsic satisfactions are possible for nurses only when the administrator is sensitive to and accountable to the nurses' dissatisfactions. Supervisors and managers need to be cognizant of their impact, as well of the impact of regulations and excessive documentation. If these challenges are ignored and allowed to outweigh the positive aspects of their work, long-term care nurses may move to other employers as the current nursing crisis leads to attractive enticements such as sign-on bonuses and higher pay with greater benefits. Nursing personnel are critical to the viability of the health and long-term care industries. These industries are labor intensive, and nursing is their largest occupational category. However, the chronic shortage of nurses demands more understanding both of the dynamics underlying the attraction and retention of nurses in particular and of the workplace more generally.

CRSO

Discussion Questions

1.   Identify the educational requirements and daily functions for licensed practical nurses and registered nurses. Discuss how educational requirements are
related (or not related) to the different daily functions.

2.   Describe the economic and ethical implications of nursing ratios in long-
term care facilities. How do you think family members view nursing ratio evidence?

3.   Review the descriptions of nurses' typical (or recent) days. What feelings
did you hear in each description? Identify differences and similarities in feelings
among home care, nursing home, and assisted-living nurses.

4.   Reasons for improving communication between and among different
healthcare settings (e.g., hospitals, nursing homes, home care services) include
not only better client care, but also more effective nursing practice. Identify
practical methods for enhancing knowledge of each others' responsibilities and
functions, as well as client information.

5.   "Long-term care nurses know their clients over time and in multiple dimensions and use this knowledge in caring for them." Describe how long-term care
nurses use this knowledge of clients in their daily nursing functions.

6.   Provide some examples of how a home care nurse's values or lifestyle may
significantly differ from that of her client. How can dispensing with her beliefs
facilitate health and caring?

7.   "Caring and connecting means providing personal recognition to seniors
and encouraging their autonomy and independence." What would you infer from
this statement?

8.   Describe teaching responsibilities of long-term care nurses other than instructing clinical tasks (e.g., changing a dressing or colostomy bag). Who, other
than clients, are being taught? What special expertise or skills are needed to
teach effectively in long-term care settings?

9.   Identify the skills and knowledge needed in supervising staff. How can supervision skills be developed in nurses in an efficient manner? Why would
nurses find these tasks particularly distasteful and thankless? How can these
tasks be made more appealing to nurses?

10. Teamwork, administrative support, and positive staff attitudes are highly
valued by nurses. How can an administrator keep her or his pulse on these values (monitor them) within an organization?

11. Consider the statement that nurses could not remember even having an entire day they felt was "good," during which the values of teamwork, administrative support and positive staff attitudes were visible. What would it take to help nurses have entire days which are "good?"

12. Home care was described as the last positive place to practice nursing. What would you infer about this statement? How can assisted-living facilities and nursing homes be changed to be viewed as positive places to practice nursing?

13. Describe characteristics of the ideal supervisor for long-term care nurses. How could these characteristics or skills be developed?

14. Both home care and nursing home nurses report feeling stressed by their large workloads. How do their workload tasks differ? What are the common elements they both face related to heavy workloads?

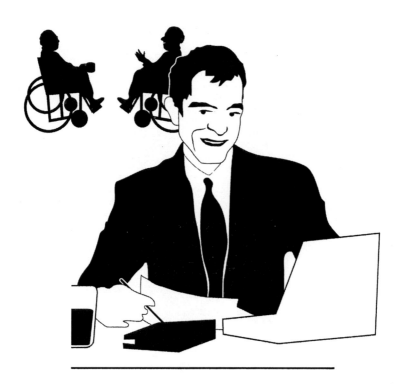

"I feel good knowing that I'm running a quality program for the seniors I love."

CHAPTER 5

VOICES OF ADMINISTRATORS

> We in long-term care are given responsibility for
> caring for the frail and sick elderly of our society.
> The order in which we set our priorities will de-
> termine how close we rise to professional status.
> Is our first concern with quality care for the resi-
> dents we serve? Do we use resident comfort and
> safety as a primary basis for purchasing and staff
> decisions? Do we feel a responsibility to provide
> life-enhancing services even in cases for which
> there is inadequate or no reimbursement? It is the
> answer to these types of questions that determine
> where we stand in the range between occupation
> and profession.[1]

Just as administrators can benefit from listening to and understanding their staff and clients, staff can benefit from considering administrators' daily tasks, challenges, and triumphs. The administrative voices in this chapter come from the senior managers of nursing homes, home care agencies, and assisted-living facilities. They include both chief executive officers and senior nurse adminis-trators, who are often called directors of nursing services. Several studies con-sidered these administrators as a group, while others separated administrators based on their specific charges. This chapter considers both the collective and individual voices of administrators identified by organizational responsibility.

Long-term care administrators yield substantial influence over their em-ployees, as well as over organizational spirit and culture. Equally important, however, administrators influence the quality of care seniors receive and nursing home inspectors find. One national study found that nursing homes with high administrative turnover had higher percentages of residents who had bed sores, were catheterized, and were given psychoactive drugs.[2] The director of nursing is especially important to residents of nursing homes. In another national study, the longer a director of nursing had worked in a home, the more residents rated their care as highly satisfactory.[3] State inspectors recognize the importance of long-term care administrators in the life of a facility and try to inspect facilities within six months of a change in either the administrator or the director of nurs-ing.

This chapter starts by describing the typical functions of long-term care ad-ministrators. Most of the challenges encountered by these administrators are similar, but the details and priorities differ. Each administrative position has been explored by core job analysis studies which have identified the fundamen-tal tasks and responsibilities professionals in these positions perform. Next, the administrators' personal and professional values are presented. The chapter ends with administrators' major challenges and dissatisfactions. As the material in this chapter will reveal, an increasing number of long-term care separate table within this chapter.

Daily Functions of Administrators

Simply put, providing quality care with limited resources is the charge of long-term care administrators. In contrast, much more detailed descriptions of administrators' tasks have become available since a congressional act mandated that their basic tasks and functions be described and updated every five years. This congressional mandate also developed a national examination that reflects nursing home administrators' primary knowledge base. This was done through a study in which working nursing home administrators identified and described their daily tasks. The first study was conducted in 1985, and now the National Association of Boards of Examiners for Nursing Home Administrators commissions a job analysis study every five years. The most recent domains of practice identified for nursing home administrators are (1) management, governance, leadership; (2) personnel management; (3) finance and business; (4) the environment: industry, laws, and regulations; and (5) resident care.[4]

Although not federally mandated, job analysis studies of home care and assisted-living facility administrators and directors of nursing have also resulted in the development of certification examinations.[5, 6, 7, 8] While licensure examinations cover basic minimum competencies, certification exams cover the familiarity with specific tasks and knowledge necessary for excellence. Certification programs and examinations are voluntary and available to administrators in all areas of the long-term care continuum. The study guides used in preparing for the examinations provide a good overview of the daily tasks and responsibilities of each position. Table 5.1 presents the major categories of competence for each long-term care administrator.

As the table on the next page reveals, the major tasks across job categories are the same: financial, organizational, and human resources management. These three duties consume the most time in an administrator's day—from 50% to 60%. Some task categories vary by setting. For example, administrators of nursing homes and assisted-living facilities perform physical environment management functions, while home care agency administrators have information management functions at their core. All administrators have some client care responsibilities.

Financial Management

Financial management tasks include analyzing financial statements and budgets along with assets and revenue management. Specific tasks include developing and evaluating the organization's budget, monitoring financial obligations, and approving and monitoring vendor contracts and department budgets. The majority of home care and nursing home executives feel that maximizing reimbursements and optimizing overall financial performance were some of their top priorities, and they spent a large proportion of their time dealing with financial matters.[9] Directors of nursing, however, do not manage organizational or departmental finances as much as they would like. Most directors felt this was due to the demands of other, more pressing, matters; although some directors of nursing felt barred from access to financial information by their administrators.[10]

Table 5.1 Primary Functions of Top-Level Administrators in Long-Term Care Organizations [a]

Nursing Home Administrators	Nursing Home Director of Nurses	Home Care Agency Administrators	Assisted-living Facility Administrators
Finance and business	Financial management	Financial management / reimbursement	Business & financial management
Personnel management	Human resources	Human resources	Human resources
Management, governance, leadership	Management, planning, reviews & rounds	Organizational planning & management	Organizational management
Physical resource management			Physical environment management
Resident care oversight	Evaluating patient care	Quality/risk management	Resident care management
The industry, laws and regulations	Handling regulations, forms, and reports	Legal / regulatory management	
	Public relations / Communication with clients & families	Public relations / marketing and community education	
		Ethics	
		Information management	

a: All functions identified in national job analysis studies[4, 5, 6, 7, 8]
Source: Data compiled by Janet R. Buelow, 2006

The amount of time spent in financial management is usually related to the size and affiliation of the facility. Nursing home administrators in hospital-affiliated facilities spend less time on financial management than administrators of independent facilities or nursing home administrators employed by multi-facility companies.[11] A study of proprietary nursing home administrators found that most administrators control four financial areas: (1) revenue source reports, (2) expense reports, (3) income statements, and (4) department work hours. Generally, administrators reviewed these reports at least monthly.[12]

Most administrators must know the reimbursement requirements of Medicare, Medicaid, and private insurance for their particular industries, as these are seniors' typical funding sources. Both nursing home and home care administrators have fairly new prospective payment systems with reimbursement rates based on a complicated mix of diagnosis and client behavioral and functional status. Administrators must monitor not only the reimbursement code of each client, but the length of service of the client in order to ensure that funding does not run out. One study of nursing home administrators found that although administrators already used a number of cost control methods, the prospective payment system (PPS) induced them to add more.[13] Within two years of the new PPS implementation administrators managed their facilities in ways that allowed them to benefit from its special features. The most popular new cost control method was maintaining a high occupancy of heavy-care (high-reimbursement) clients.

Although nursing home administrators closely monitor Medicaid revenues, assisted-living facility administrators typically do not have access to Medicaid reimbursement in their states; alternatively, the reimbursement is so low that the ALF does not accept it. Nevertheless, these administrators also need to keep facility census up for financial health. Assisted-living facilities have a longer cycle, and clients and families spend an average of four months deciding to move to such a facility. Thus, assisted-living facility administrators spend more time marketing and developing a broad referral base to keep their facilities financially viable.[14]

Human Resources Management

Personnel and human resources management includes recruiting and hiring staff, as well as training, evaluating, and disciplining employees. Each administrative position identified different functions within this domain. However, directors of nursing seemed to have the most responsibilities.[15] Nursing directors identified coordinating and scheduling staff, dealing with staff conflict, and evaluating adherence to quality standards and regulations as the most time consuming and constant challenges. Other personnel tasks the majority of nursing directors dealt with regularly were recruitment and staff absenteeism.[16] All administrators, whether of home care facilities, nursing homes, or assisted-living facilities, recognize staff retention as their primary human resources challenge. This extremely difficult problem will be discussed in more detail later in the chapter.

Several nursing home administrators stressed that choosing key staff members wisely is vital. One nursing home administrator said that she tried to select staff who valued good service and cooperation because technical expertise can always be taught.[17] Another nursing home administrator explained how he focused on developing department directors and supervisors in fulfilling his human resources development functions.[18] He tried to keep supervisors thinking they were there to do the very best possible job of taking care of residents; redefining their roles from "playing policemen" to role modeling for staff members. Similarly, a former nursing home administrator urged her managers to build trust and a positive collaborative culture with their staff. She pushed her managers to see the world through their employees' eyes, stressing the necessity of understanding their feelings.[19]

Management

Organizational management functions include planning, organizing, leading, coordinating, and controlling. A large part of these functions occur in the process of simply "wandering around." For a home care administrator, "wandering around" is not possible, but consistent, friendly telephone calls are. Specific activities vary from one organization to another, as well as, from time to time, in the same organization. A study of home care administrators found that small- and medium-sized agency administrators prioritized operational duties. In contrast, administrators of large home care agencies prioritized fiscal tasks above operational duties.[20] Nursing home administrators who have hired many nursing directors identify organizational management functions as most important for this position. Specific skills they look for are in the arenas of leadership, people and relationships, and effective decision-making. A direct aspect of organizational management decision making is visioning. One director claimed that she must solicit ideas on how to do something better, to "offer more, improve customer service, and measure the outcome." For example she must envision how a decision is likely to affect the patient, caregiver, employee, payer source, and the financial bottom line.[21]

Physical Environment Management

Managing a physical environment is one function home care administrators do not perform, but with which nursing home and assisted-living administrators deal every day. Although certain tasks are necessary regardless of the age of the facility, generally speaking, the older the structures, the more time an administrator spends on environmental management. Physical environment management tasks include creating and maintaining a safe and healthy structure with approved fire, emergency, disaster, and resident security plans in place. Emergency repairs and preventive maintenance are also administrative tasks. The majority of administrators also mentioned providing a home-like setting as one of their environmental tasks.[22]

Resident / Client Care

To provide quality long-term care services, administrators need a basic knowledge of the aging process and related conditions and diseases. They also need to know the client care demands for their particular long-term care organization. Common administrative tasks in this area include conducting periodic care plan reviews with clients and their families, ensuring compliance with appropriate medication and health care policies and procedures, and upholding clients' rights to determine their own care.

Clinical care is not most administrators' original domain. Although many home care administrators have a nursing background, many others rely on their directors of nursing to inform and advise them regarding clinical care issues.

During informal communication and in focus groups, long-term care administrators often admit a need or desire for more clinical knowledge. One comprehensive study found that nursing homes with an administrator with a nursing background had fewer survey deficiencies than did homes with an administrator without a nursing background. In fact, the three strongest administrator characteristics predicting survey deficiencies were short tenure, little time spent with residents, and lack of a nursing background.[23]

Regardless of clinical background, long-term care administrators believe they should be regularly available to their clients and their clients' family members. Both nursing home and assisted-living facility administrators indicate taking a lot of time to talk and problem-solve with clients. One administrator with a non-clinical background felt that he contributed to his clients' general health by facilitating his facility's resident association.[24]

Managing Legal and Regulatory Mandates

Long-term care is a highly regulated service industry. Administrators must keep up with specific industry statues and regulations, and general health care laws. Additionally, because long-term care is very labor intensive, administrators must know applicable labor laws and regulations. Antitrust and state tax laws, too, are a concern for administration.

In one survey, home care executives claimed that knowing and dealing with regulations was not only critically important but also more time consuming than any other administrative task.[25] Directors of nurses, too, claimed that they were very involved in ensuring adherence to reimbursment and quality assurance regulations.[26] In summation, all long-term care administrators are involved with managing the enormous number of regulations that guide the industry.

Marketing Functions

Each long-term care administrative position involves some marketing activities. However, the majority of administrators considered marketing duties part of management tasks. Home care executives and assisted-living administrators both identified a stronger marketing emphasis in their jobs than did nursing home executives. Specific tasks identified included market analysis, segmentation strategies, and product differentiation.

All in all, long-term care administrators' duties and responsibilities cover a broad range of knowledge areas and managerial skills. One home health director said, "At any moment, my role changes from coach, to cheerleader, spectator, player, go-fer or referee."[27] Administrators must anticipate, meet, and exceed a diversity of needs in conducting the business of long-term care.

Values and Satisfactions

Administrators at skilled-nursing homes, assisted-living facilities, and home care agencies all indicate that their top priorities are facilitating a high quality of life for clients and providing quality care.[28] These seem to be the overriding professional values of administrators. A high-quality life is defined as living in a comfortable environment where one receives respect, has personal control over his or her own care, and gets both social and health needs met. One assisted-living facility administrator said, "Quality of life is customer focused and market responsive, not regulation driven."[29] Quality care as opposed to quality of life generally involves supporting staff activities that maintain each individual's highest physical and psychosocial functioning. Examples of such activities are preventive skin care, range-of-motion exercises, and friendly conversations with staff and others.

In a national survey of nursing home administrators and directors of nurses, "treating residents with dignity" was overwhelmingly rated as the most important component of quality of life care.[30] Another priority that over 60% of administrators and directors of nurses valued was "promotion of residents' rights." This meant ensuring that seniors had self-determination including the right to be informed and the right to be free of reprisal if one complained or reported a problem.[31]

Home care administrators seemed to agree with these priorities. In a survey identifying organizational and leadership factors related to excellent care, home care administrators were most concerned with quality of life issues, which consisted of facilitating the best living environment, maintaining daily living activities, and ensuring coordinated services.[32] Also, as part of these priorities, home care administrators were very concerned with obtaining program funding for health promotion activities.

Data on administrators' personal values are difficult to find as surveys rarely ask about them directly. Nevertheless, a few job satisfaction surveys and turnover studies identified some consistent values and expectations that influenced administrators' satisfaction.[33] Two values were powerful enough to influence nursing home administrators either to describe serious dissatisfaction or actually leave their profession if they were not actionable in the organization: the ability to make a difference through their decisions or leadership skills and job autonomy.[34] Two values were also found in a survey of new nursing home administrators as reasons they were attracted to their jobs: (1) they wanted to help people, and (2) they wanted to reform or improve nursing home care.[35] Although these altruistic values were identified only among nursing home administrators, administrators in other long term services are assumed to hold these or similar personal ideals, too.

Dissatisfactions and Challenges

Just as with direct care assistants and nurses, the nation is experiencing a shortage of long-term care administrators. Nursing home administrators' turnover rates average 20 to 30% and several states report that fewer administrators are choosing to renew their licenses.[36] In addition state boards report a steep decline in administrators joining the field as identified by the number of new applicants taking the licensing examination. These findings indicate dissatisfaction among administrators, and this indication is supported by several surveys of long-term care administrators that identify high rates of dissatisfaction.

Certainly all categories of long-term care administrators include both satis-fied and dissatisfied individuals. However, it has been primarily nursing home administrators and directors of nursing who have been studied, and therefore, little is directly known about home care administrators' satisfaction. Still, based on more general measures, it appears that the majority of assisted-living admin-istrators are fairly satisfied with their positions.

Job dissatisfaction and turnover among nursing home administrators are definitely linked. One study of Texas nursing home administrators found that administrators who were more likely to leave their jobs early claimed that their primary reason was "job dissatisfaction."[37] The dissatisfactions most frequently identified were poor quality care in their homes, insufficient staffing, and feel-ings of powerlessness to improve conditions. Other dissatisfactions noted by administrators planning on resigning were poor benefits, pay, and promotions; lack of recognition and support; as well as a high number of routine, non-administrative tasks.

A study of nursing home administrators in North Carolina found similar dissatisfactions. In this study, nursing home administrators thinking of leaving their jobs were dissatisfied with the leadership style of their bosses, a mismatch between personal and organizational values, and lack of opportunities for growth and advancement.[38]

Two studies of nursing home administrators found a relationship between administrative turnover and poor performances on state surveys.[39] In both stud-ies, administrators with short tenures had more survey citations than did other long-term facility administrators. These administrators also exceeded budgets and had high staff turnover.[40]

Two studies of directors of nursing identified additional dissatisfactions. Both surveys found that directors were very dissatisfied with their salaries; one wrote that her duties and responsibilities were comparable to those of hospital-based nurse managers, yet her salary was not commensurate.[41]

Other areas of dissatisfaction among directors of nurses were the amount of paperwork and the lack of benefit packages, especially retirement benefits.[42] The second survey of directors of nurses found dissatisfaction with the lack of ad-ministrative support, specifically in budget allocations, in staffing ratios for weekends and holidays, and in opportunities for continuing education.[43] Nursing directors wanted money for in-service education and off-site training experi-ences. They also wanted to attend at least one regional or national conference a year and to receive paid subscriptions to health care journals that focused on senior care.

Directors of nursing are also not staying very long in their positions. In one state survey, 75% of the nursing homes had had up to five new directors of nurs-ing in the last five years, while 11% had had between six and twelve nursing directors during this time. The nursing home administrators (their bosses) be-lieved the top reasons directors of nursing left their positions were not enough pay and too much responsibility, stress and burnout, and increased regulations.[44]

Professional Challenges

Problems described by administrators can be categorized as client care issues, managerial challenges, and social problems. Client care issues are related
to seniors' needs and preferences, as well as family members' concerns. Managerial challenges include problems of staff quality and availability, appropriate
leadership styles, and cost control strategies. Social problems encompass nursing homes' poor image, which limits the number of people willing to even consider working in the field. Tough regulations, coupled with low government
reimbursement practices, are also considered societal challenges.

Client-Centered Care

Recognition of the need for client-centered care is emerging among administrators. Joy Calkin and Judith Ryan were the CEOs of the two largest national
chains of long-term care organizations in the late 1990s (Extendicare and The
Evangelical Lutheran Good Samaritan Society, respectively). International
search firms selected them for the right combinations of skills and knowledge to
lead these long-term care organizations. Interestingly, both CEOs have nursing
backgrounds, and in interviews both projected a personal, resident-centered approach to running their organizations. Both of these executives voiced an over-
arching vision of how a long-term care system should work, with clients leading
the way.[45]

Assisted-living administrators, more than other administrators, identify client and family concerns as a constant challenge. Knowing every client and his or
her family members was often mentioned as an essential responsibility of a successful assisted-living administrator. Several assisted-living administrators
pointed out that assisted-living facilities have fewer direct-care and indirect-care
workers, so administrators must be available to clients on a consistent daily basis. In assisted-living facilities, the administrator is the one who has to have his
or her door open all the time. As one said, "I spend a lot more of my time problem-solving with residents and family members. When I was in the nursing
home setting, I typically had a social worker on my staff who handled many of
these issues."[46]

A related challenge is anticipating what seniors and their family members
want. In most assisted-living facilities, and in some other long-term care facilities, seniors themselves pay for services, and administrators must meet and exceed their expectations. One assisted-living administrator said, "I used to spend
a lot of time thinking about how to keep my nursing home out of the regulatory
firing line. Now I spend a lot more time thinking about the private paying customer's needs and how to meet them."[47]

Nursing homes' directors of nursing often referred to their work as "quality
auditing" or as monitoring each client's care to ensure that it was the most appropriate and of the best quality possible. In a study of top-quality nursing
homes, nursing directors perceived quality auditing as their most time consuming work role.[48] Quality assurance actions often involved clinical monitoring,
setting up special routines and policies, and teaching and modeling client-
centered behaviors.

Home care administrators described a different challenge in the area of client-centered matters—teaching staff that clients are in charge. These administrators noted that many of their staff had come from nursing homes where they were in charge of setting residents' schedules. In the words of one administrator, "In a home care setting, the balance of power shifts from staff to consumers, and the client's living space is where he or she can exercise control. The staff must treat seniors as tenants in their homes, rather than as residents in an institution."[49] This is completely different from a nursing home, where nursing staff are on their own turf and seniors must comply with staff preferences. In home care, seniors can set their own schedules, choose their food, and even reject medical and nursing advice. This is quite different from a nursing home or even an assisted-living setting with set daily schedules and plans.

Home care administrators rely on seniors to notify them if care is not to their liking. In one study of top-quality home care agencies, administrators were given brief scenarios of typical client problems (e.g., worker-client clash, poor worker skills, client prefers different time of day for visit) and were asked how they would discover such problems. In all scenarios, the majority of administrators relied on their clients to inform them of problems or potential challenges.[50]

Staff Recruitment and Retention

Long-term care administrators identified staffing as one of their most critical challenges. The current high turnover rates and the shortage of available staff are endless operational problems, and some also acknowledge the harsh employment conditions of frontline staff. As one nursing home administrator said, "One of the things that you can't be prepared for until you're actually in the situation is running an organization that relies very heavily on frontline caregivers who are not given the pay or the respect that they deserve. The lack of equity and social justice really smacks you in the face." [51]

According to the American Health Care Association, many nursing homes are forced to turn patients away and even close facilities due to the lack of available staff. These shortages are occurring at the registered nurse, licensed practical nurse, and other professional levels, but the shortages are most severe for the care assistant positions. Staff turnover problems exist in every type of long-term care organization. In a national survey of over 800 home care administrators throughout the nation, 56% said they were having difficulty recruiting and or retaining RNs and another 48% indicated problems in recruiting and retaining assistants or aides. When asked to name the single most important factor contributing to the nursing shortage, most administrators mentioned low wages.[52]

Home care administrators described similar problems only with more complications from staff turnover. One primary frustration was their inability to raise salaries to stay competitive with hospitals because of Medicare caps. Agency after agency commented on the inhumane system that permits only poverty wages and no benefits for homemaker-home health aides. Another central complaint is documentation requirements. A national study found that home health nurses spend over 50% of their time allocated to patient visits completing documentation.[53] many nurses take their paperwork home in order to prevent it from cutting into patient care. Administrators worried that the primary draw to home care nursing, one-to-one nursing, is being undermined by massive documentation requirements. One home care administrator wrote that staff nurses were forced to complete "mountainous paperwork at the cost of patient care time, only to see their efforts wasted as the denials for care kept rolling in."[54]

In this same national study, home care administrators were asked to check the factors that they believed contribute to the RN shortage. Increased paperwork showed up with the greatest frequency (72%), followed by noncompetitive salaries (69%). Other causes, cited by about 30% of the administrators, were weekend work, no advancement, poor image, and minimum benefits. In the comment area of the survey form, administrators wrote that retention had not been as much of a problem as recruitment until area hospitals had begun raising salaries. Factors contributing to homemaker-home health aide shortages were low wages (60%), transportation problems (38%), poor benefits (35%), no advancement (34%), poor role image (29%), and inadequate training (24%).[55]

Assisted-living administrators are also concerned about staff recruitment and retention.[56] Karen Wayne, president of the Assisted-living Association stated, "To compete, we need to spend as much time selling to potential staff as [to] potential residents."[57] Administrators are urged to analyze the competition for employees in their areas. The average hourly wage for an assistant should be compared to retail-sales wages and factory work. Benefits and upward mobility should be understood as part of the draw to these jobs and compared to those offered to care assistants. Clearly, when unemployment is low, potential direct-care assistants easily find less demanding, higher paying jobs. Competition sources also differ by region. For instance, where gambling is legal, casinos draw many applicants away from assisted-living facilities.

The staff shortages in long-term care are most severe for care and nursing assistants. The U.S. Bureau of Labor predicts that direct-care positions will be among the top ten occupations with the largest and the fastest job growth rates over the next decade. Currently, with 1.25 million active caregivers, the United States will need an additional 600,000 caregivers by 2011. This trend in job availability is offset by a national unemployment rate of 2.9%, which means there are just not enough applicants to fill vacancies. In addition to low unemployment, the long-term care industry faces an average direct-care worker turnover rate of 93%, compared to the average labor turnover rate of 10%. In other words, care assistants are leaving their jobs much faster than the industry can recruit them. Furthermore, even if the unemployment rate increases, and more people seek these jobs, many may not fit the profile of a typical care assistant. Demographically, 89% of care assistants are women aged 25 to 54, most are low-income, and many are ethnic minorities. Over the next 30 years, the number of seniors who need direct care will only increase, while the numbers of U.S. women 25 to 54 will steadily decrease.[58]

Staff Management Skills

Many long-term care administrators suspect that the nurses employed in long-term care settings contribute to the problem of care-assistant retention. One administrator stated, "The graduate nurse does not receive sufficient training in administration and supervision. These are her primary responsibilities when employed in a nursing home. I have lost what I believed to be good aides because my supervising nurse is not sensitive to the difference between occupational and educational supervision."[59] A survey of directors of nursing found that although they agreed that their nurses needed some human resource expertise, many admitted that they themselves needed more skills in this area. Nurse administrators rated their interest high and competence low in human resources skills. Priority education areas were motivating staff, managing staff turnover, managing problem employees, and professional staff development.[60]

Some directors of nurses believe part of the problem lies with administrators' drive for profitability. A nursing director wrote that when she told facility administration that budgeting cutbacks were hampering her staff's ability to provide adequate care, she was told that the ownership had a fixed level of profit that had to be achieved.[61] She thought that a legislative solution requiring a minimum staffing ratio for facilities is needed. In a national survey, 85% of nursing directors agreed that while minimum staffing is not the ideal, at this time it is necessary. A staffing ratio based on need of care would be the ideal scenario, but currently the necessary information is not available; so nursing directors support a minimum staffing ratio based on number of clients. Many nursing directors reported a lack of authority to staff their facilities based on levels of needed care. They indicated that even though they and their staff are responsible for subacute care (fresh hip replacements, tracheotomies, etc.) they have not been "allowed" to supplement their staff.[62]

Leadership

The leadership skills required of a long-term care administrator are very complex. While hospital administrators are concerned primarily with business and financial operations, long-term care administrators must also supervise staff and conduct direct interactions with seniors and their families.[63] These extra responsibilities may be the reason several studies have found a direct relationship between administrative leadership style and quality of care.

One study of the ten nursing homes judged as giving the best overall quality of care found that without exception, the nursing administrators' attitudes, commitment, and interpersonal skills were highly respected by their staff. Directors of nursing in these high-performance homes were respected for their commitment and caring attitudes. This commitment was evidenced in their dedication to high standards and in the enormous enthusiasm and effort they put into their work including working outside official hours and at home. They were often influential in professional organizations and caregiver support groups. In these homes, the nursing directors were perceived to be the final authorities and ultimate sources of control in all matters related to resident care.[64]

Like nurses, nursing directors want management and leadership training. In one Michigan survey, over 50% stated they needed management education. Specific areas of training identified as needed by 90% to 100% of nursing directors were communicating with superiors and subordinates, motivating staff, managing conflict, dealing with difficult people, conducting performance evaluations, and disciplining subordinates.[65] In one state survey of both nursing home executive officers and their nursing directors, both indicated the need for management education for themselves. Interestingly, the executive officers thought less of their nursing directors' skills than the directors themselves did. In this study, 71% percent of the nursing directors believed they had the necessary management skills to succeed in their positions, while only 49% of the chief executive officers thought the nurses had the necessary skills. The top three areas identified as most important were human relations skills, basic management knowledge, and facility monitoring.[66]

In surveys and focus groups, administrators made many general recommendations regarding how to recruit and retain staff effectively. Recommendations included creating a positive work environment; maintaining high values and standards; and providing job security, adequate salaries, and benefits. Recommendations for retaining care assistants included enhancing their perceptions of self worth and value as part of the team, creating career ladders, providing more responsive supervision, and creating ownership in their evaluations.[67]

Cost Control

With the introduction of prospective reimbursement systems, first in nursing homes and then in home care agencies, cost control has become a growing challenge. One study surveyed administrators before and after a significant change in the state's reimbursement policy to determine the effects on their managerial practices. Nursing home administrators were making extensive use of cost control methods at the time of the first survey, but they made substantial additions and modifications following the new payment system's introduction. They increased cost control methods by about 30%, with the majority of these changes using profit maximizers, instituting new cost controls, and initiating new policies based on reimbursement incentives.[68]

This survey asked administrators to review lists of cost control strategies (e.g., monitoring expenditures, comparative pricing, centralized group or bulk purchasing) for each of their cost centers. The average percentages of the specific cost control measures for each cost center varied from 69% to 90% before the new reimbursement system. After the new system, the percentage of cost control measures for each center ranged from 74% to 95%. The top cost control methods prior to the reimbursement change were in (1) medical and nursing supplies, (2) plant operations and maintenance, and (3) dietary services. Two years after the new system, the most significant increases in cost control methods were in medical and nursing supplies, dietary services, laundry services, housekeeping services, and administrative and management methods.[69]

One of the primary measures found after the new system started was a substantial increase in the number of heavy-care Medicaid patients (from 42% to 73%). A popular cost control response was to start using special incentive features of the new reimbursement system; almost half of the administrators stated they had retained savings through these provisions. The most popular incentive activities were maintaining a high occupancy rate and a stable proportion of heavy-care Medicaid patients.

An examination of current case mix-adjusted reimbursement policies suggests that this system rewards administrative cost control. Nursing homes that increased the proportion of Medicaid residents and eliminated excess beds experienced greater profitability gains during the beginning phase of this reimbursement system. (Prior to this reimbursement reform, having a heavy-care resident population was related to lower profits.)[70]

A study conducted before the prospective reimbursement system was instituted examined which management practices kept cost per patient day down and profit per patient day up. Seventy randomly selected nursing homes (both proprietary and nonprofit) were studied over a two year period using both administrators' perspectives on their cost control practices and their annual reports filed with state departments of social and health services. The results showed that higher profits per patient day were related to the use of more management control practices. Also, the total number of years an administrator had managed a facility was positively associated with profits per patient day. Higher profit per patient day was also associated with smaller nursing homes.[71]

Negative Image

The negative image of long-term care administrators is a constant challenge, especially for nursing home administrators. One nursing home administrator said, "Our biggest issue is the image and stigma of who is served and who are nursing home administrators....There is a lack of appreciation for the work, the workers, the level of sophistication needed....The negative press is not only demoralizing, but also causes administrators to leave their profession or to not consider long-term care as a career."[72] Similarly, a director of nursing said:

> I don't like to use the term "nursing home." It's like rest homes...they were always these little dingy homes. . . .People usually know I'm a nurse and they usually know I'm a director of nursing. And when they ask where I work, I tell them I am the director of nursing in a 180-bed skilled-nursing facility. I don't say I am the director nursing in a nursing home, because immediately people wonder, What kind of a person are you?[73]

One long-term care administrator noted that he had received many negative comments when he had made a "crazy" jump from hospital to long-term care administration: "It was viewed a second-class career."[74] There is no doubt that this negative image exists and is felt among long-term care professionals.

Regulatory Requirements

Nursing home administrators must keep abreast of changes in regulations which include licensure and certification requirements governing nursing homes, labor laws, Occupational Safety and Health Administration (OSHA) regulations, and the Life Safety Code. They must then implement programs, procedures, and surveillance mechanisms to maintain compliance. All these regulations and compliance programs demand constant monitoring and are considered major stressors. As Charles H. Roadman II, president of the American College of Healthcare Administrators, stated:

> Increasingly I hear from my members that they're disheartened....Administrators say they are not doing what they signed up to do; they're consumed by a mountain of regulations and spend much of their day deciphering onerous regulations....I know they'd rather spend more of their time providing hands-on management and care.[75]

Nursing directors also experience great stress from dealing with regulations and often feel that many of the regulations are in conflict with their professional judgments.[76] Directors feel the survey process is negatively focused, punitive, and misdirected, and believe that they are often meeting the needs of the surveyors rather than promoting quality resident care. One survey respondent pointed out that issuing citations and deficiencies is adversarial and counterproductive to meaningful change. Although an appeal mechanism was in place to contest citations, the cost was often prohibitive. Therefore, facilities often just paid the fines that were imposed while the issues remained unresolved.

Directors of nurses also express frustration at being watched and criticized, and some resigned because of the anxiety-provoking nature of the survey process. One said, "In no other branch of nursing do you have the media, surveyors, and people outside of the industry trying to tell you that you did a bad job."[77] This nursing director admitted that regulations were necessary but added that regulatory bodies needed to provide education and assistance in implementing and adhering to regulations, an approach that empowers rather than oppresses.

Many assisted-living administrators have expressed fear about the federal or state regulations that might be imposed as they admitted more disabled seniors to their facilities. All were afraid that regulation would be punitive, rigid, and excessive. As one assisted-living administrator reflected on the nursing home business, he noted that the state is in an adversarial role, as they control dollars which keeps pay low. Then often regulators have a difficult attitude during survey visits. He said it would be sad if this happens to assisted-living facilities.[78]

Administrators often acknowledge that regulations and accreditation standards are part of an insurance plan to ensure quality care. They realize that they must play the regulation game to get reimbursement, but in focus groups they came up with recommendations for better approaches.[79] Some recommendations included (1) assessing the competency of all staff, (2) developing certification for first-line managers, (3) establishing outcome-oriented goals and objectives communicated throughout the organization, (4) developing critical pathways using standards from the American Nurses' Association and the Agency for Health Care Policy and Research, and (5) monitoring customer satisfaction (of physicians, patients, vendors, etc.). They also suggested that organizations develop good relationships with educational and voluntary agencies to enhance their resources and analyze quality care patterns and trends. Finally, administrators recognized that to ensure quality services they had to maintain a minimum data collection system and analyze for trends.[80]

Conclusion

As the studies that open this chapter reveal, long-term care administrators must have both managerial and financial skills, and a solid understanding of the clinical and psychosocial actions that support older adults in our society. They not only oversee health care services, but also are responsible to meet social, mental, and rehabilitative client needs. In addition, these administrators are often responsible for the safety of their clients' living situations, whether in nursing homes, in assisted-living facilities, or in clients' own homes. Consequently, long-term care administrators have the full range of administrative and managerial tasks of similar-sized organizations and the responsibilities for many private lives, responsibilities which used to be addressed within the family.

This unique combination of responsibilities is further complicated by the huge impact long-term care administrators have on their staff who care for vulnerable, needy individuals but who are often deprived themselves. The government's responsibility to ensure quality care for vulnerable individuals imposes multiple regulations and additional responsibility. These regulations are derived from both health care concerns and societal and cultural expectations, and are often viewed as solely the long-term care administrators' challenge.

The voices of these administrators provide insight not only into the long-term care industry, but also into our society. Great demands and expectations are placed on administrators of long-term care organizations. After listening to their perspectives and those of their staff, one cannot help but question the expectations we have placed on them. The final chapter of this book, "Successful Programs," responds to all of these perspectives and is provided to end on an inspirational note. There are several programs run by administrators which seem to acknowledge and respect client and staff voices. Administrators of these programs have not only listened but responded to the voices within their own facilities. First, however, the next chapter compares the four voices of long-term care.

CR80

Discussion Questions

1. Clearly, administrators do not provide direct clinical care, so why do you think there is a correlation between administrator turnover and the number of residents with bed sores?

2. Financial, organizational, and human resources management tasks consume over 50% of a long-term care administrator's day. List tasks identified for each of these three areas. Then identify where differences may lie among nursing home, home care, and assisted-living administrators.

3. Staff retention is identified as the primary human resources challenge of all administrators. Why do you think this is so? How can it be avoided?

4. Since an administrator with a nursing background receives fewer survey deficiencies, what can a non-nurse administrator do to insure good survey results?

5. Why do you think both home care and assisted-living administrators identify stronger marketing emphasis in their jobs than do nursing home executives?

5. Top personal satisfaction areas for long-term care administrators are facilitating high quality of life and ensuring quality care. How can administrators see these satisfaction areas fulfilled?

7. Several reasons were identified for nursing home administrators to leave their jobs. Identify those reasons that seem easiest to change versus those reasons that may need more systematic changes. Support your answer.

8. Do you agree with the reasons nursing home administrators gave for why their directors of nurses left their positions so frequently (not enough pay, too much responsibility, stress and burnout, and increased regulation)? Do some of these reasons contradict each other?

9. There is a trend in long-term care organizations towards client centered care; yet, home care administrators noted that they had the challenge of "teaching staff that clients are in charge." Furthermore, many of their staff came from nursing homes where the staff set seniors' schedules. Compare the challenges administrators from home care agencies and nursing homes face in the area of client centeredness. How would programs focused on developing client centeredness differ from those that are not?

10. One of the primary challenges recognized by all long-term care administrators is staff recruitment and retention. Identify at least three reasons administrators gave for this constant challenge. For each reason, provide a few suggestions administrators could try. Why do you think these suggestions have not been used or why they have been used but have not worked?

11. Leadership and management skills were identified as challenges, especially for directors of nursing versus those in other administrative positions. How would leadership skills differ among nursing director, nursing home administrator, home care agency executives, and assisted-living administrators?

12. The last three challenges identified by administrators were cost control, dealing with negative images, and keeping up with regulations. How do these compare to the primary challenges of staff recruitment and client centered care? What are possible relationships among these challenges?

CHAPTER 6

COMPARISON OF VOICES

"The implications of these findings indicate that administrators who believe they understand and communicate effectively with their residents may indeed not perceive the residents correctly as frequently as 70% of the time."[1]

Long-term care organizations present a complicated challenge both for seniors who are being served and the caregiver who is serving them. The purpose of this chapter is to identify the similarities and differences between the caregivers and seniors served within long-term care systems. Daily activities, personal and professional values, as well as challenges are reviewed for each stakeholder. These perspectives are then compared to identify shared aims and common needs.

For this chapter several comparative studies were reviewed. Some studies involved both seniors and staff within home care and nursing home organizations. Others compared voices of nursing assistants and nurses. These caregivers provide intensive care to seniors and must be able to work together as a team. Their perceptions highly influence the care they provide and their abilities to meet needs of the seniors they serve. Last, comparative studies of administrators and their staff in nursing home and home care agencies are included.

Personal Values

The voices of seniors, regardless of where they reside on the long-term care continuum, are remarkably consistent. Seniors value their independence and want control over their lives and the services they receive. Living in safe surroundings is important to them, as well as compatibility with their primary caregivers. Seniors want staff who will listen to them and respond to their preferences and who are trustworthy. These are the most basic wishes of seniors, regardless if they are using home care services, assisted-living services, or residing in nursing homes.

Seniors place high value on several specific staff characteristics. Nursing staff who are cheerful and do not bring their problems to work are displaying the most fundamentally desired characteristics. Also, having enough staff so the senior feels that help is available when needed is very important.

Specific services mentioned by seniors as important are housekeeping tasks and a health professional who is available by phone to check out an unusual health symptom or concern. For seniors in congregate settings, the meal options are very important. Not only do they want choices, but they also want tasty meals and some flexibility for meal times and table partners.

After listening to the seniors, we listen to nursing assistants, the staff closest to seniors. Frontline staff overwhelmingly value hard work and ambition in their personal lives. They are proud of being helpful and capable in helping their families as well as the seniors for whom they care. These values are not only voiced, but are also witnessed in assistants' personal lives, as many have pulled themselves and their families out of difficult circumstances and on to more stable lives. Most frontline staff members have little psychological or fiscal support and often are the heads of household for dependent youth.

Two studies compared values of seniors living in a nursing home to those of nursing staff and administrators working in the nursing home. The first study asked nursing staff and administrators to rank ten values they thought were most important to the seniors for which they cared.[2] Then the seniors themselves ranked these values. Seniors ranked the ten values very close together: family and visitors, clean and comfortable surroundings; good food; caring staff; feeling useful; affection; religious activities; social activities; flexibility in daily schedule; and privacy, respectively. Administrators and nursing staff ranked seven of the ten values significantly lower than seniors, with the greatest contrast being between administrators and seniors. Clean and comfortable surroundings, feeling useful, religious activities and flexibility in daily schedule were the values not recognized by administrators and nursing staff, while having family and other visitors and good food were correctly identified as top values for seniors.

The second study compared the ratings of nursing staff and seniors in ten different nursing homes, some with very poor ratings and some with excellent ratings.[3] Regardless of the quality of the homes, ratings by nursing staff were more favorable than the seniors' ratings, but were only significantly different in poor quality homes. In poor quality homes, seniors believed that they received less respect, communication, response from calls, and concern from nursing staff. In addition, they also believed the nursing staff did not like their work. In better quality homes, seniors thought the nursing staff was more supportive and encouraged more self sufficiency among the seniors. The three descriptors by which seniors discriminated poor quality nursing homes from excellent nursing homes were: feeling that nursing staff treated them with respect, feeling that nursing staff liked their work, and having at least one staff member who was special to them.

How do beliefs of seniors receiving home care services differ from how nursing staff view them? One study in this area used nursing documentation to compare to seniors' voices during telephone interviews.[4] Note that comparisons may lack some validity as nurses may document only issues which are reimbursable. In this early study only seniors receiving an average of four home care visits per week had significant differences between nurses' documentations and seniors' descriptions of their health problems. Seniors reported their most common problems as fatigue, sleep disturbances, appetite changes, and ambulation problems. Nurses, however, rarely noted these problems; rather, they documented seniors' most common problems as knowledge of and skills in doing prescribed treatments, as well as not clearly understanding their medications.

In another study of seniors just discharged from the hospital and starting home care services, differences were again seen between the reports and ratings of nursing staff and those of seniors.[5] In this study, seniors rated themselves better in activities of daily living (walking, eating, etc.), as well as medication management than their nurses' documentation indicated. This data indicates that better communication between nurses and seniors is needed, along with better research methods in this area.

In summary we see that those closest to seniors have a general understanding of seniors' values and challenges. On the other hand, many specific aspects of care and preferences are not recognized by nursing staff. Additionally, many long-term care staff do not realize how much seniors value their independence, control over their day or services, and some flexibility in scheduling or activity by their primary staff caregiver. Likewise, frontline staff or nursing assistants may not be understood as valuing the ambition they have shown throughout their personal lives and work.

Daily Activities

How do the daily functions of long-term care staff compare? Looking at daily functions of both the frontline staff and nurses of long-term care organizations, several aspects of their jobs overlap. Both groups of staff members provide direct care to seniors with hands-on functions. Also, both provide psychosocial care which incorporates the caring, loving, human aspect of service; apparently, staff members also struggle with burnout and related attitudes that result in less than caring behaviors.

Nursing assistants describe the types of daily care they give as many of the activities of daily living such as bathing, dressing, and assistance with toileting. They describe doing for seniors what they can no longer do for themselves. Home care assistants, too, perform assistance with activities of daily living, but also offer the tasks of light housekeeping which seniors can no longer comfortably perform. Much of the care all nursing assistants provide is physical work that includes lifting seniors who are immobile; sore backs or other injuries are common, especially in situations in which the numbers of staff are insufficient. This includes helping a person into and out of the bath, assisting them in washing, perhaps moving furniture so that the senior is more comfortable, and even reaching tough places in the home or room from which the senior may need things and that he or she has waited for the assistant to get. Nurses describe their direct care as less physical, but as equally direct in working with seniors. Direct care from nurses includes distributing medications, changing dressings, and performing physical assessments. Direct care from nurses also includes care which is invisible care to seniors, such as calling a physician, adjusting care plans, and checking on the seniors' insurance coverage.

Psychosocial care is given every day by both nurses and nursing assistants. This would include interpersonal exchanges between staff and seniors given either during functional care activities or just in passing each other during the day. Both nurses and nursing assistants felt they gave encouragement and comfort to seniors when needed. Observations of both nurses and nursing assistants did reveal that they gave a great deal of sympathetic care and were nearly always kind despite outbursts or moodiness on the part of seniors.

Custodial care is defined as negative psychosocial behaviors found in a small percentage of nursing assistants and nurses, especially by staff who were burned out. Custodial care includes acting in a paternal manner, such that staff opinions are considered to be better than seniors' opinions. Burned out behaviors are caused by emotional exhaustion, and it often leads to depersonalization of seniors. Ignoring or avoiding seniors who are asking for help are examples of depersonalizing behaviors by staff. Several studies comparing attitudes of nursing assistants and nurses have found that nursing assistants have the lowest empathy level and highest custodial orientation towards seniors.[6, 7] Nevertheless, both nurses and nursing assistants seem to be experiencing moderate levels of burnout in the areas of emotional exhaustion and depersonalization.

Several studies observed assistants treating seniors with impatience or irritation, while other studies found nursing assistants and nurses being irritated by seniors while helping them. Also, it was found that nurses expressed more empathy and responsiveness to seniors wanting autonomy than did assistants. Still, several studies recorded burned out nurses and nursing assistants speaking about how they could depersonalize their jobs and prevent seniors from asking for something or talking about something the nurses and nursing assistants did not want to hear. One daily activity of nursing assistants, mealtime assistance, seems to have much associated custodial care. In one study, it was found that only 5% of the time, the assistants asked the senior he or she was feeding if he or she wanted a particular food before offering it.

Supervision is an activity recognized by all staff as unsatisfactory, yet only nurses identified it as one of their daily activities. Their supervision was usually over nursing assistants or other frontline aides, and the nurses freely admitted they did not like to supervise, nor did they feel qualified to do it. As one nurse said, someone needed to supervise the assistants, but it was a thankless job. Nursing home managers noted that conducting performance evaluations and giving constructive criticism were tremendous challenges for the nurses. Some administrators voiced concerns that nurses' inadequate supervision skills were driving frontline staff away.

Daily activities of administrators differ significantly from frontline staff and nurses. Administrators of nursing homes, home care agencies, and assistant living facilities all seem to have similar duties that can be clustered into categories such as financial, human resources, and organizational management. Additionally, they all are responsible for monitoring and assuring quality care. Furthermore, all administrators need to keep up to date with various safety regulations, as well as insurance regulations. Administrators of assisted-living facilities and nursing homes also have physical environment management as part of their daily activities. Obviously, none of the administrators' daily activities overlap with the daily functions of nurses and nursing assistants. As Table 6.1 reveals, team members' activities are so different that an understanding and appreciation for each long-term care staff member must be deliberately and thoughtfully provided.

Table 6.1 Comparison of Daily Activities of Long-Term Care Team Members

Frontline Staff	Nurses	Administrators
Functional Care	Direct Care	Financial Management
Psychosocial Care/ Custodial Care	Caring and Connecting	Human Resources Management
Mealtime Assistance	Teaching and Coaching	Organizational Management
Work Styles: Efficient & Novice	Supervision	Structural Management
Extra Initiatives	Burnout behaviors	Client Care Oversight
Abusive and burnout behaviors		Managing Regulations
		Marketing Functions

Source: Data compiled by Janet R. Buelow, 2006

Satisfactions

An ideal organization is one in which individual staff achieve a sense of satisfaction through their work and are working towards a common purpose; we have hope that it will be the right purpose. In other words, staff should feel proud of their work and feel valued for their labor. Also, staff work should be directed towards the priorities of the clients served. By listening to long-term care staff and administrators talk about what they truly value about their work and how their work is meaningful to them, several commonalities are identified. These professional satisfactions are presented in Table 6.2.

The ability to help seniors is extremely meaningful to all those working in long-term care organizations. Nursing assistants, nurses, and administrators all voice great satisfaction in serving seniors with quality services and loving care. Administrators, true to their backgrounds, value the opportunity to make a difference in seniors' lives through their decisions and applied leadership skills. This value for administrators is strong enough that those who do not feel able to provide it are more likely to leave their jobs. Both high quality of life for seniors and excellent clinical care are the outcome and services which administrators identify as within their realm of accountability. Quality services involve treating seniors with dignity while facilitating the best living environment, maintaining daily living activities, as well as ensuring that clients have control over their preferences. The ability to make a difference in the lives of seniors is very important. Some new administrators seek to foster reform of the system upon which seniors are forced to rely.

Nurses and nursing assistants identify similar values in their own words. Nursing assistants identified a sense of contributing valuable services which society needs. They mentioned that they could be making more money in the local fast food restaurant, but felt proud that in their current jobs they were helping people who needed them. Similarly, nurses valued "making a difference" in others' lives.

A personal relationship with someone was also important to assistants. The assistants often viewed themselves as family to the seniors they cared for and saw themselves as a nurturing family member. This caring is revealed in the many ways in which assistants went beyond their duty in caring. Giving special occasion cards and small gifts, and completing extra chores were often witnessed as acts by assistants intended to help their senior clients. Nurses identified the opportunity to care for whole persons—physically, socially, and psychologically. They valued the time they got to spend with their senior clients in a long-term care setting, as well as the ability to help seniors at home deal with health problems in the reality of their own homes.

Professional values which keep a person working when things are rough are important. With long-term care staff all teammates seem to have similar satisfactions and professional values. Despite different daily tasks, they each recognize the positive aspects of their jobs and can reinforce with each other the value of their jobs and labor.

Table 6.2 Comparison of Team Members' Satisfactions

Frontline Staff	Nurses	Administrators
Give valuable services	Make a difference in people's lives	Provide leadership which insures that seniors are provided a high quality of life
Close relationships with seniors	Caring for the whole person	Leadership to enable better / good quality care
Autonomy *	Autonomy *	Autonomy**

* This satisfaction was identified by home care staff only.
** This satisfaction was identified by nursing home administrators only.
Source: Data compiled by Janet R. Buelow, 2006

Challenges

Constant work challenges and problems can wear individuals down and at times even make the satisfactions of work seem to disappear. Many challenges experienced among frontline and nursing staff are similar—poor salaries, inadequate supervisors, unmanageable workloads, and poor staffing ratios as well as lack of professional respect. Each of these challenges is frustrating to frontline staff and nurses, and many are directly related to one of the greatest challenges frustrating administrators: recruitment and retention of quality staff. Other challenges recognized by multiple team players in long-term care are the tremendous burden of regulations, leading to demanding documentation requirements for nurses. Last, the emerging challenge of changing the culture of care to client centeredness is identified by many administrators.

Work overloads are probably one of the biggest challenges the frontline staff and nurses face on a daily basis. Frontline staff members regularly grumble about their workloads and the number of seniors they are assigned to care for each day. In interviews, assistants often mentioned that they went home feeling bad about what they did not finish doing for their clients. The challenge of workload overload was voiced much differently from nurses than from assistants. The nurses primarily stated that they had the mandatory amount of staffing, but it just seemed that the seniors needed more care and, therefore, their work was never done. Home care nurses, too, did not complain about workloads as much as not always getting everything done for their clients. These things included the actual visit and care, new admissions, documentation, driving, phone arrangements, and staff meetings. Nurses spoke of feeling frustrated when they are denied more visits with their clients and must assume their clients are safe at home. Feelings in this area sometimes lead to negative feelings towards administration. Nursing assistants often stated they felt that administrators were not responsive to seniors' needs by keeping the staffing so low that the seniors' needs could not be met. Nurses voiced similar feelings of frustration with not being able to accomplish all the care needed, and directed some of their frustration towards administrators of their organizations.

Poor supervisory and managerial skills in leaders were found as challenges by all three long-term care team members. Furthermore, many nursing assistants identified their supervisors and general management as their strongest points of dissatisfaction. In fact, poor supervisory relations were the most common reason given by assistants for leaving their jobs. In some studies, administrators were witnessed treating nursing assistants with contempt by undercover researchers acting as nursing assistants. Many nurses also had negative feelings toward supervisors. This was true for nurses in all long-term care settings. Nurses wanted a supervisor who could support and respect their opinions and hard work, with a clear understanding of their jobs and its challenges, and who looked out for the needs of both the clients and staff. While nursing directors identified needing managerial skills and welcomed training in this area, administrators identified lack of leadership skills among their nursing staff as a challenge in their work. Administrators identified lack of leadership as a significant challenge which they felt led to other problems. They believed they had lost good frontline staff due to charge nurses with insensitive supervisory skills.

Disrespect is a common complaint voiced by all team members; however the disrespect was felt to come from different parties. Nursing assistants stated they felt disrespected by clients' family members, nurses, and administrators. Family members were mentioned by both nursing home and home care assistants as often challenging them with accusatory statements or making unrealistic demands. Several assistants voiced the feeling that family members assumed they neglected their relatives and wanted families to know that they were doing their best under very heavy workloads. Disrespect by their supervisors was often mentioned when assistants discussed their everyday work. Lack of respect by supervisors was one of nurses' most common complaints, too. These feelings are important, as several studies found that negative feelings toward supervisors are the primary component driving nurses and nursing assistants to leave their jobs. Physicians also admit to disrespecting nurses in nursing homes and that they believe these nurses' professional judgment is inferior to that of hospital nurses. However, just the opposite is felt by home care nurses, with nurses reporting collegial relationships with many physicians. Administrators felt the negative press of nursing homes was disrespectful of staff and administration and contributed to the fact that many individuals are not even considering working in long-term care.

Documentation demands due to increasing and changing regulations were challenges both nurses and administrators voiced. Nurses in both nursing homes and home care mentioned that necessary documentations had grown tremendously with shifts in Medicare and cost control goals. Nurses in home care agencies see ten to twenty page documents per patient that need completion, while nursing home nurses have just as lengthy documents needing completion every few months with their clients. Nurses often confessed to trying to outwit the regulations to benefit their clients. They would make sure just the right amount of improvement was witnessed so that their documentation would ensure continuing Medicare coverage. Administrators felt frustration with keeping abreast of changes in regulations required to keep licensure and maintain certification status. They voiced great frustration with spending the major part of their days deciphering regulations and ensuring that all details were complete. Nursing directors felt much of the regulator survey process was negatively focused and felt they were often meeting the needs of the surveyors rather than promoting quality resident care.

One of the last challenges mentioned by nursing assistants and nurses is dissatisfaction with their income. Home care assistants added to this dissatisfaction the insecurity of not being able to rely on a steady income because their pay is so contingent on clients staying in their homes. Financial security for nursing assistants included high rates of uninsured health care for themselves and family members. Furthermore, assistants seem to be losing health coverage more rapidly than other American workers. Although this challenge was heard from all staff it has not been found as a significant cause for leaving one's position as have some of the other challenges voiced by long-term care workers. Salaries are lower for RNs in nursing homes than hospitals; this seems to be a long time reality. Interestingly enough, the salaries for LPNs are just the opposite, with these nurses making slightly more in long-term care settings than in hospitals.

Administrators spoke of some of the same challenges their staff recognized; however, they also had some dissatisfactions that are unique in their positions— changing a clinical culture to a more client focused one and controlling ever rising costs. Knowing every client and his or her family members was often mentioned as an essential responsibility of long-term care administrators. This is not the case in other areas of health care administration. Another aspect of the challenge of being client focused is teaching staff that clients are in charge and that the staff is there to serve them. The old way of running care, with staff being in charge, has to be changed; often, that change is difficult to accomplish.

Long-term care administrators have always made extensive use of cost control methods in managing their long-term care organizations, but with new regulations they are employing substantially more, using profit maximizers and initiating new policies that are based on reimbursement incentives. Along with cost control, administrators identified the constant challenges of staff recruitment and retention as the most critical of the challenges they faced. High staff turnover problems exist in every type of long-term care organization and administrators recognize the challenge of being dependent on frontline caregivers who are not given the pay or respect that they deserve. They expressed frustration with not being able to raise salaries to be competitive with hospitals due to Medicare caps and with requiring mountainous paperwork of their nurses. Some administrators mentioned that they needed to spend as much time selling to potential staff as to potential clients. Often, lack of leadership skills were blamed for their second most common challenge. Administrators feel their supervisors are often to blame for not being able to keep good assistants as their lack of proficient leadership drives these individuals away.

In summary, the challenges long-term care staff face are numerous and overlapping. The top challenge among all long-term care administrators is staff recruitment and retention. Getting and keeping high quality staff seems to be a continual challenge, as does maintaining the organizations' financial solvency in light of government regulations. These administrative challenges seem to be passed on to the staff, as their primary challenges are poor staffing ratios or work overload, feeling unappreciated and insecure financially. It is unclear if each party is aware of the others' challenges. Gaining empathy from team members may be beyond most staff members as they struggle to meet client needs.

Table 6.3 Comparison of Team Members' Challenges

Frontline Staff	Nurses	Administrators
Financial security	Low wages	Change to client-centered culture
Supervisors & management	Managerial inadequacy	Staff recruitment and retention
Poor staffing ratios => work overload	Work overloads	Leadership & management skills
Indignities & disrespect	Disrespect	Cost control
Inadequate training	Document requirements	Negative image & disrespect
		Regulations

Source: Data compiled by Janet R. Buelow, 2006

Conclusion

Communication within long-term care organizations is rarely all that it can be. With the range of individual values and background experiences mixed with the pressure of constant physical and mental demands, one can understand how so many different perceptions can impact the process. This lack of clarity and ease in communication can contribute to team members not working together as well as could be possible in caring for seniors.

It is clear that all team members are working hard and that their overall purpose and professional joys are congruent. All staff members seem to want to provide the best quality care possible. All feel bad when the best care is not provided and seniors are left with less than optimum care.

Nevertheless the direct care team members, nursing staff and nursing assistants, are the ones who experience most of their challenges on a personal level. They are the ones who seem to be running with direct functional care tasks and the mentally challenging tasks of caring for individuals who are struggling at this time in their lives. These team members feel at a very visceral level both the satisfaction of helping someone and the even stronger pain of seeing a hurting individual neglected due to the physical impossibility of their being able to be two places at one time. This experienced pain must be directed somewhere and it seems to be directed up within the organization to administrators.

Fortunately, administrators have satisfactions that are similar to those of the frontline staff and nursing staff. They sincerely want seniors to have a high quality of life and to receive loving care. However, their daily work takes them away from witnessing whether quality care and services are constant in seniors' lives, and some administrators admit discomfort with less than desired care. The primary challenges of administrators then are focused on more tangible symbols and the tasks of their position, most notably, gaining and keeping their nursing and frontline staff.

In listening to administrators list their daily tasks, it is clear that often their work is more than one individual can achieve, especially considering systemic challenges. Still, it is just as clear that with more communication, real listening and understanding among team members, that better care for seniors is possible. Frontline staff members need to understand the daily challenges administrators are facing. As well, administrators must see and understand the daily challenges and psychological pain frontline staff face in their jobs. With real recognition of each other's challenges, teamwork and real problem solving may be possible.

CRSO

Discussion Questions

1. How do the most common values of seniors, independence and safety, compare to your most important values? Do you think age impacts one's priorities?

2.   Having compatible caregivers is a priority value of seniors needing long-term care services. How would you describe this value and how does it fit with the values of independence and safety?

3.   Frontline staff's top two values are hard work and ambition, with ambition being defined as capable of helping. Compare the top values of seniors and frontline staff. How do they compare and fit with each other?

4.   In one study it was found that administrators and nursing staff did not fully recognize seniors' values of clean and comfortable surroundings, feeling useful, access to religious activities, and flexibility in daily activities. Suggest specific ways administrators and nurses can recognize these values within a nursing home or assisted-living facility. How can they recognize these values within home care services?

5.   In one study it was found that in poor quality nursing homes, the nursing staff did not treat seniors with respect and did not seem to like their work. Additionally, none of the individual staff were special to the seniors. How do these three aspects of care interrelate? Create an improvement plan that addresses these three aspects of care within a nursing home.

6.   Why do you think seniors receiving home care services view their health challenges differently than the home care nurse reports them? Suggest a different method to study seniors' perceptions and the perceptions of nurses in this regard. What could cause such differences in perceptions of health needs?

7.   How are the daily activities of nurses and nursing assistants similar? How are they different? How do these staff members work together to support seniors' needs for independence and safety? How can their methods be improved to support these preferences of seniors, as well as seniors' need for compatible caregivers?

8.   Several studies recorded burned out nurses and nursing assistants speaking about how they could depersonalize the seniors in their jobs and thus prevent seniors from asking for something. This depersonalization was done as a response to their burned out feelings. What can staff and administrators do to prevent depersonalization? How can depersonalization be stopped quickly when detected and what type of monitoring system can be set up to detect depersonalization as early as possible?

9.   It seems that not only is depersonalization a problem, but supervision is also a problem in long-term care. Identify several training programs available in your area. How do they focus on preventing or addressing burnout and the consequent depersonalization of seniors?

CHAPTER 7

SUCCESSFUL PROGRAMS AND STRATEGIES

> "Imagine a nursing center staffed with nursing
> assistants who have stayed with you for years and
> yet maintain a fresh, enthusiastic perspective
> about their job. Imagine newly graduated RNs
> who choose long-term care as the setting of
> choice and have years of experience in working
> with the elderly. An impossible dream? Not with
> the implementation of ....."[1]

It seems only right to close this book by considering programs responsive to the voices presented in previous chapters. Many excellent programs address some of their concerns, and this closing chapter examines successful programs and strategies in long-term care organizations. In this context, programs are considered successful if they meet some of seniors' expressed values and preferences or address frontline assistants' and nurses' identified job challenges and dissatisfactions. Successful programs focus on seniors' health, functional and psychosocial needs, and on ensuring that clients control most aspects of their own care. Programs that promote staff dignity, professional values, and growth, with the intention of promoting job satisfaction, are staff retention programs that are highly related to client dignity and to staff professional growth and job satisfaction; they would also be considered successful.

A review of the literature revealed a plethora of program descriptions. The first criterion for inclusion in this chapter was having goals to improve matters significant to seniors, assistants, or nurses (e.g., staff satisfaction, rather than profit margins, or increasing client control, rather than increasing Medicare, Part A, services). The programs noted in this chapter are considered the most generalizeable to other organizations, where they should yield similar outcomes.

However, many excellent strategies and programs in long-term care organizations have not undergone empirical evaluation. Some of these programs provide a great starting point and ideas for enhancing services. Programs with promising ideas for enhancing services are described in this chapter. Any programs implemented will need "fine-tuning" to fit the specific individuals, history, and culture of a given organization.

In reading through the descriptions of programs in this chapter it is important to keep two points in mind. First, most programs described had multiple positive outcomes, regardless of their success in meeting the original goals. For example, permanent-assignment programs for care assistants were intended to improve assistants' turnover rates, and, while this goal was not always met, such programs did result in improved care and senior satisfaction. Hence, it is important to keep an open mind regarding both a given institution's particular concerns and the many possible outcomes of a given program.

A second consideration is that while individual strategies can be statistically related to positive outcomes, their actual contribution to any given outcome is usually very small, often less than 10%. However, using many such strategies in conjunction, such as part of a package of programs, greatly increases the likelihood of positive outcomes. In fact, the greater the number of programs implemented, the more likely positive outcomes become. It is recommended that no program be implemented in isolation, but rather as part of a package of different strategies. Examples of such packages for both home care agencies and nursing homes are presented, along with individual program descriptions.

Client-Focused Programs

Research clearly shows what works and what does not work in creating exceptional client services. What does not work are motivational speeches, one-day customer service training, and posters or button paraphernalia. The single most effective way to create exceptional client service is to develop a culture wherein staff members are totally committed to meeting and exceeding client and family expectations. Such a culture includes the following elements: (1) shared values, norms, beliefs, and ideologies which are clearly and consciously focused; (2) committed senior management; and (3) skill-training programs.[2] Examples of client-centered programs developed in a variety of long-term care organizations follow. Although staff appreciated some programs more than others, each program described successfully improved some aspect of seniors' lives. Each program's essential components and outcomes are presented.

The Wellspring Model [3]

Eleven Wisconsin not-for-profit nursing homes aligned in 1994 to create the Wellspring Model. Wellspring culture values and respects not only the individual senior, but also each employee, regardless of department or function. The belief underlying the model is that few nursing assistants work only for pay; rather, assistants are attracted to work in nursing homes because they want to make a difference. Wellspring focuses on line staff in all departments, showing them the difference they can make on a daily basis.

Outside evaluators of the Wellspring alliance have conducted extensive pre- and post-program surveys, as well as open interviews, with seniors and staff. They found that Wellspring nursing homes have more satisfied seniors and staff, higher senior immunization rates, fewer bedfast seniors, lower rates of restraint usage, better preventive skin care, less use of psychoactive medications, less senior incontinence, and fewer tube feedings. Additionally and significantly, Wellspring homes had the same staff ratios as other nursing homes in the state but demonstrated significantly better staff retention.

Much of the Wellspring model is based on the premise that when an organization has knowledgeable staff, those staff members take pride in their daily work. Furthermore, when members of the management team take time to help line staff understand how they impact organizational outcomes, the staff are more receptive to change.

Since 1998, six other groups of nursing homes throughout the nation have formed alliances and have been working with Wellspring to replicate the model in their organizations.[4] The Wellspring Model program components that these organizations implemented over a two-year period are found in Table 7.1. A key determinant of the program's success is the commitment of middle managers, and especially staff nurses, to mentoring front-line staff. Both management and line staff have education modules to complete, but the management module is given first. This module is designed for top and middle managers, and takes place over three days with the objective of teaching managers to become coaches, mentors, and enablers of necessary culture change. Areas of focus include staff empowerment, change, coaching techniques, and problem-solving strategies. A personality profile is administered to staff members to facilitate teambuilding. Upon completion of this module, managers must return to their facilities and assess organizational readiness for the Wellspring program.

Following this evaluation, the clinical education modules are provided next. They are based on nationally defined best practices in specific areas of elder care. These modules are led by a Geriatric Nurse Practitioner (GNP) and the consulting clinicians (e.g., dieticians, physical therapists) assigned to care resource teams from each facility. A care resource team has the responsibility of ensuring that each organization is utilizing best practices. During the education module, these team members are administered personality profiles and educated in building self-directed teams, essentials of proper documentation, infection control, senior rights and communication, along with the best practices of their particular clinical modules. The teams report to management within their facilities and have six months in which to implement enhanced care before an evaluation is conducted. Throughout the program, data is collected and team members, with the coordinator and GNP, identify challenges and plan changes designed to improve care.

All alliances are doing well as measured by higher immunization rates, fewer bedfast seniors, lower rates of restraint usage, more preventive skin care, less use of psychoactive medications, less senior incontinence, fewer tube feedings, and more varied diets than in comparable homes—all with the same staffing.

The Caring Touch [5]

The Caring Touch program was implemented as a pilot study in an Illinois nursing home. The aim of this program was to communicate an attitude of caring to seniors through appropriate touch, improved listening, and empathic understanding. A Caring Touch is defined as a one-to-two minute interaction which involves both physical touch and verbal reassurance. It is not the context, duration, or location of touch that is the key; it is the attitude and meaning of touch in practice. Voice, tone, volume, effective listening, and the degree to which the body relaxes during the interaction communicate a message of caring and concern.

Table 7.1 Wellspring Model Components

1	Create an alliance of 5 to 12 facilities within two hours' driving distance
2	Top administrators begin meeting monthly
3	Facilities begin permanently assigning staff to groups of seniors
4	Facilities establish coordinator position (RN) to attend all meetings and education modules
5	Facilities recruit geriatric nurse practitioner (GNP)
6	Management Module Education (3 days)
7	Facilities establish "care-resource teams" for each clinical module, with 5 to 6 line staff per facility
8	Clinical Education Modules (2 days)
	Geriatric physical assessment
	Elimination/continence
	Skin care
	Nutrition
	Dementia care
	Falls prevention
	Restorative care
	Palliative care (recommended, not required)
9	Care resource teams make facility changes (policies, education, and process)
Quarterly	GNP visit each facility to evaluate data and check with care-resources teams

Source: Data organized by Janet R. Buelow, 2006

To begin the program, assistants participated in ten one-hour training sessions in which they were taught to clear their own inner spaces, to listen to and receive from seniors, and to understand nursing home seniors' inner worlds. The first training sessions developed listening skills. This meant listening without giving advice, passing judgment, or rushing in to fix anything. The second sessions taught assistants to clear a mental space from the clutter, worries, and problems of their personal lives. Next, assistants learned to appreciate seniors' experiences. They role-played being disabled seniors and practiced entering the external personal space of another person – moving slowly and gently into each other's spaces, giving their partners time to receive them. Last, assistants learned how to let seniors reach out to them. Receiving care was very difficult, but it is a necessary skill because seniors often want to give something back to their caregivers.

For the next three months assistants noted in seniors' charts when they provided Caring Touch. During this time, the number of Caring Touches received by each senior ranged from approximately one to six per week.

Program outcomes were measured by comparing seniors and staff on floors with Caring Touch to those on floors without it. The Caring Touch floors started with less healthy seniors who required more medications. After nearly three months, these seniors maintained their level of satisfaction and morale and required fewer medications. The floors without Caring Touch maintained morale, but satisfaction declined, and use of psychotropic medications remained constant.

The most positive effects of this program could be seen among the care assistants. More than a year later, they were still enthusiastic about Caring Touch. They felt it had had a positive impact on their lives and had changed the way they viewed seniors. The assistants who had gone through the training had significantly lower turnover and tardiness rates than did other assistants in the same homes. They reported higher morale and satisfaction and said that a new team spirit had been created among them. They felt their relationships with seniors had greatly improved.

Outstanding Assistant of the Quarter [6]

Another example of a client-focused program is entitled "Outstanding Nurse Aide I of the Quarter." This program was developed to recognize care assistants' exceptional performance. Each quarter the program started anew, and assistants could elect to join it at the beginning of any quarter as often as they liked. However, they were dropped if they received a reprimand or missed more than two weeks of work.

There were two segments of the program: interventions and rewards. Interventions were created from assistants' answers to the question, "What tasks go beyond accepted practices to outstanding practices with seniors?" Forty tasks were identified and categorized on an evaluation checklist. The categories included grooming, bathing, bowel and bladder care, feeding, comfort, compassion, social interaction, attitude toward facility, care planning, and charting. Examples of grooming tasks were cutting/cleaning nails between weekly baths, applying lotion throughout the shift, and shaving seniors between weekly baths. Feeding tasks included conversing with seniors, offering fluids between meals, and encouraging slow feeders to take extra nutrition. Initiative tasks included cleaning drawers, arranging clients' rooms, and helping coworkers after an assistant's own work was done.

Rewards were designed to give assistants the highest visibility at a low cost to the facility. Rewards included (1) a recognition lunch at the facility attended by the administrator and other managerial staff; (2) a certificate of achievement presented at the luncheon; (3) a photograph of winners displayed in the main lobby; and (4) a free chicken dinner certificate donated by a local fast-food vendor.

Observation and evaluation scoring of the participating assistants was done by the charge nurses and senior care assistants. The most significant outcome of this program was increased job performance. This may have been due to the survey tool alone: many assistants expressed surprise during the program evaluation at all the possible tasks they had not thought of doing before. Also, participating assistants who suddenly increased their job performance put pressure on non-participating assistants to do the same.

However, assistants noted several negative outcomes. First, there seemed to be an increase in bickering among assistants. Instead of engendering teamwork, the program unintentionally promoted competition. Voluntary dropouts became more frequent as the program progressed due to the participants' perception that their scores did not reflect their actual work performance. Also, assistants felt the entire staff was watching them, and they expressed anger and embarrassment if they did not receive an award. Last, the administrative time required by the program was prohibitive. In the end the program developers wondered if a unit program would have been more beneficial than an individual one. However, the assistants were very negative about this idea.

The Household Project[7]

The Household Project was started in a continuing care retirement community in Oshkosh, Wisconsin. The program's purpose was to determine how a change in physical environment and management approach that was teamed with empowered staff would affect seniors' satisfaction and quality of life as well as caregiver productivity.

Physical environments were changed so that eight seniors lived in a house with four private and two double rooms arranged around a light, airy living space that included a living room and a farmhouse kitchen. Seniors dined together at every meal and participated in a variety of activities. The staff was a consistent set of employees who received 30 hours of training and functioned as a team.

An evaluation revealed that seniors' mobility, socialization, and satisfaction had greatly improved. Interviews with seniors and families were quite positive. The families observed significant positive changes in seniors' functioning, happiness, cognition, and activities. Family members seemed more involved and treated other seniors as extended members of their own families. One daughter said, "Before my mother moved to the Household, she never communicated with the staff or with other seniors, and she never wanted to leave her room. In the Household, she is rarely in her room, preferring to be out in the pleasant and quiet living area, playing cards or talking to the staff." [8] Another family member stated that the biggest change she noticed was in the caregivers and how they really worked as a team. A revealing comment from a senior was, "Now when I say my prayers at night, I thank God that there's a place like this for me to live, and a place like this for someone to come to when they need it." [9]

Senior-Centered and Senior-Driven Community [10]

This program is similar to the Household program, but it also serves disabled seniors. The Northern Pines Community in Minnesota is a licensed nursing home divided into three groups: a community of 16 seniors who provide some of their own care; a 16-person community of seniors with cognitive challenges; and a community of 8 seniors who require extensive care. Prior to creating their senior-centered and senior-driven facility, the nursing home sent 150 stakeholders (administrators, nurses, frontline staff, and senior spouses) to visit 17 other long-term care facilities known for their senior-centeredness. The objective was to transform the home into a senior-centered and senior-driven community utilizing the information gathered during these visits.

The first move towards senior-centeredness was physical renovation to create three home-like environments; removing department silos and bringing decisions closer to the seniors; and involving all parties in design, implementation, and ongoing learning. Other key components were (1) a blended workforce; (2) team decision-making meetings; and (3) career ladders for the staff. The blended workforce component consisted of all frontline staff receiving training in each others' roles. As cross-training was completed, frontline assistants received pay raises and began to spend about 20% of their time cleaning rooms and cooking meals. Frontline workers were paid to participate in weekly decision-making meetings with seniors and managers. The frontline staff also had 10 caregiving areas to learn; with completion of each, they received a small per-hour raise. Three other areas of training and responsibilities were offered nursing assistants, so they could make even more money and had opportunities to be community liaisons. Evaluations revealed steady decreases in staff turnover and improvements in quality of care. Quality improvement measurements included a decrease in medication errors and infection rates, as well as a significant slowdown in clients' weight loss. Senior clients and their family members gave the program high satisfaction scores. Stories of improvement included one senior who started walking again, and others who began to play musical instruments they had long neglected.

The Client-Directed Model for Home Care Agencies [11]

This next model of care was developed in California home care agencies that serve low-income seniors. It offered a client-directed model (CDM) of care and compared it with the traditional home care agency model. In the traditional model, agencies hire, train, and coordinate nursing staff. In the CDM model, all of these responsibilities—recruiting, hiring, and supervising nursing staff—are delegated to clients. Home care assistants can be anyone including family members.

The program's evaluation process included telephone and home-visit interviews with clients and staff. Overall, CDM clients reported more positive outcomes than did traditional home care clients. Statistically significant differences were found in how empowered CDM seniors felt compared to their traditional home care counterparts. CDM clients were also more satisfied with the technical and interpersonal aspects of services and with their quality of life. They reported greater feelings of safety with their assistants and fewer unmet service needs.

Staff evaluations were not quite as positive. Traditional nursing staff reported more positive emotional states and experienced less worry about client safety than did CDM assistants. However, CDM assistants reported more positive relationships with clients and more comfort with assertive client roles. Job satisfaction was essentially the same among both groups.

Quality of Life Committees [12]

This Quality of Life program's goal is to engage seniors, families, and staff to evaluate and improve the quality of life within their facility. Standardized tests of how people perceived the nursing home and how they would like it to be were completed by 60% of all seniors and staff. Seniors wanted more responsibility and self-direction and improved physical comfort, privacy, and sensory satisfaction. They valued opportunities to express feelings and concerns, influence the institution, and to not be unduly restricted by regulations. Staff, too, gave priority to seniors' independence and physical comfort, but staff felt there should not be expressions of feelings and concerns or anger and criticism. These survey results were shared with seniors, family members, and staff. Social workers met systematically with small informal groups, discussed assessment findings, elicited reactions, and invited people to join problem-solving committees. Three committees were formed, one each of staff, seniors, and family members. Each committee used data to identify problem areas, examine opportunities for and obstacles to change, and develop feasible plans of action. Committees were required to communicate and work with others in their constituency. Goals and projects were defined with each committee. The staff committee consisted of management and line personnel and examined physical environment, increasing orientation aides, and improving the staff lounge.

The senior committee addressed needs of new seniors and fire safety. They formed a subcommittee to welcome new seniors and a self-help group on nursing home concerns. They also hosted receptions for staff and seniors. With strong support from the social worker, they regularly surveyed seniors and worked with the results to get specific information. Generally, the senior committee was concerned with removing barriers to communication between seniors and staff.

The family committee was formed for the most severely impaired seniors. Their major goal was to strengthen the liaison between families and the home. A bulletin board was displayed to exchange information, and a family meeting was arranged at which department heads discussed their roles and functions, and physicians discussed trends in drug therapy. At the end of the program, committee members reported important gains in an increased sense of affiliation and satisfaction in contributing to the nursing home's quality of services.

Carted Dining [13]

Mealtime is an integral part of seniors' daily lives, and being in control of what and when they eat is vital. Using a cart for breakfasts is a simple way to offer choice and foster independence. Seniors were given menus to fill out in advance, which were used to stock food carts. A breakfast cart was stocked to serve approximately 80 seniors without interruption. Minimal training was given to nursing assistants and dietary staff prior to program implementation.

This last program is one of the simplest, but it addressed an important concern of seniors and had excellent outcomes. This breakfast-on-the-cart program reduced senior weight loss and consumption of commercial supplement drinks while increasing average intake. Interviews with seniors showed a 15 percent increase in satisfaction with breakfasts. Furthermore, mildly to moderately impaired seniors seemed to like the increased ability to make choices, and even severely impaired seniors made choices with help. Family satisfaction increased as well; family members were often found assisting their relatives to make selections from the menu.

Staff-Focused Programs

Quality of Work Life Programs in Home Care Agencies[14]

The largest and undoubtedly most significant study of home care programs involved eleven agencies in four geographical areas: San Diego, New York City, Milwaukee, and Syracuse. Home care agencies included both subsidiaries of national and regional for-profit chains and nonprofit agencies. Program components in each home care agency were developed from combinations of suggested strategies with the intent to improve the assistants' worklife quality, job satisfaction, and propensity to stay with their employers.

The suggested strategies were (1) enhanced training; (2) support for supervision (professional or peer); (3) wage increments; (4) supplemental benefits (vacation, sick leave, and/or health insurance); (5) increased job stability or guaranteed hours; (6) status enhancements such as uniforms and name badges; and (7) staff promotions. Each agency created its own package of strategies, and many agencies shaped strategies to their particular circumstances. The number of strategies adopted ranged from four to six, and all programs included supervisor support and status tokens. For evaluation purposes, each home care agency was compared to a similar agency that was used as a control for comparing staff outcomes.

Selected strategies and agency turnover rate improvements are presented in Table 7.2. From the table, it is clear that the more strategies that were implemented, the more staff turnover rates improved. Costs ranged from $165 to $2,500 per person, per year. Further investigation of these programs revealed many intangible benefits, such as heightened staff self-esteem, increased general morale, and increased organizational loyalty among the nursing staff. Additionally, many case managers believed there was an improvement in quality and continuity of care.

Multi-Strategy Programs for Nursing Homes[15]

This large study of nursing home multi-strategy programs invited all homes in the Minneapolis / St. Paul area with staff turnover rates of 70% or higher to participate. Each nursing home agreed to report detailed turnover data quarterly for two years, attend semi-annual meetings, and implement at least five new strategies in their program. Nineteen homes remained in the study for two years, and of these, 7 were very successful (reducing turnover rates between 39 to 76%), 5 were moderately successful (reducing turnover rates between 14 and 27%), and 7 were unsuccessful (their turnover rates either decreased minimally or actually increased).

Table 7.2 Agency Strategies and One-Year Turnover Rate Change

Location	Training	Supervisor Support	⇑ Wages	⇑ Benefits	Job Stability	Status Tokens	Possible Promotion	Rate Change
NYC	X	X	X			X		11%
San Diego	X	X		X	X	X		21%
Milwaukee		X	X	X	X	X	X	44%
Syracuse		X	X	X	X	X	X	44%

Source: Data organized by Janet R. Buelow, 2006

From Table 7.3, it is apparent that the more strategies were implemented, the more staff turnover rates improved. Successful homes used more than twice as many strategies as unsuccessful ones. The five most significant strategies: (1) increased supervision of new employees; (2) supervisory training; (3) revised personnel policies; (4) increased recruitment efforts; and (5) avoidance of personnel pools.

These last two studies (as well the Wellspring Model) support the thesis that only one or two strategies cannot have a significant organizational impact. Multiple and appropriately chosen strategies, however, can have a significant impact. Additionally, no one package of strategies can ensure successful outcomes. Each area has individual variations in local labor markets and agency-specific employment conditions. In addition, the long-term acceptance and success of a program often depends on participation in the design and ownership of new strategies.

Orientation Program

Several new orientation programs have been implemented and evaluated by nursing homes and home care agencies. Most of these programs targeted care assistants for improved job satisfaction and retention, while a few included goals of specific client outcomes, such as improved client satisfaction, fewer incidents of agitated behavior, or lower infection rates.

Three examples of effective orientation programs are presented. Two programs, one in a nursing home and one in a home care agency, targeted improved staff turnover rates. The other program targeted specific caring responses of staff and was found to have improved turnover rates as well. All three programs utilized similar components, such as mentoring, individual testing, and corresponding improvement plans, but each program also employed unique approaches that added to staff and client satisfaction.

Table 7.3 Turnover Rates and Strategies of Most Successful vs. Least Successful Nursing Homes (x = most successful homes and ✔ = unsuccessful homes)

Turnover Rate Changes Over Two Years	76%	50%	44%	40%	40%	10%	9%	6%	6%	1%
Implemented Strategies	17	17	13	17	10	10	6	2	0	0
1. Improved salaries, benefits, and bonus	X	X				✔	✔			
2. Enforced policies	X	X		X						
3. Replaced NAs with LPNs	X	X		X						
4. Altered schedules	X	X		X		✔	✔	✔		
5. Employee committees	X	X	X	X		✔	✔			
6. Employee recognition	X	X	X	X		✔				
7. Hired HR director	X	X	X	X						
8. Increased orientation	X	X	X	X	X	✔	✔			
9. Increased in-service	X	X	X	X	X					
10. Primary nursing	X	X	X	X	X					
11. Increased staff	X	X	X	X	X					
12. Exit interviews	X	X	X	X	X	✔	✔	✔		
13. Revised personnel policies	X	X	X	X	X	✔				
14. Increased recruitment	X	X	X	X	X	✔				
15. Supervisory training	X	X	X	X	X	✔				
16. Increased supervision	X	X	X	X	X					
17. Avoidance of personnel pools	X	X	X	X	X	✔	✔			

Source: Data organized by Janet R. Buelow, 2006

The first example comes from a Pennsylvania nursing home that used nursing staff involvement and peer mentoring as key components to its care assistant orientation program.[16] For each new care assistant hired an experienced assistant facilitated ten days of orientation materials and for the next three months worked side by side with the new person. This peer mentor facilitated better knowledge of job-related tasks and provided access to a close, supportive peer group.

Nurses were also very involved in this program. Starting on the first day, the floor supervisor met with the new person, overlooked her plans, and then checked in daily. RNs supervised the daily orientation, attended monthly evaluations, and advised the floor supervisors on improving new employees' performance. The RNs also gave self-written tests that new orients took at the end of each shift. Care assistant mentors were compensated for their orientation work with an increase in hourly wages and a different color uniform to distinguish their status. They were also given cash bonuses four times throughout the year, as long as the new person remained employed.

Another approach that increased staff retention in many nursing homes in New York state is the Growing Strong Roots Peer Mentoring Program.[17] Experienced assistants received six to seven hours of peer-mentor training off-site and three separate three-hour sessions called mentor booster sessions to share mentoring successes and challenges and to suggest solutions to problems. Mentoring was viewed as a supplement to, not a replacement for, usual staff training. Each mentor maintained an active relationship with a peer for at least four weeks, with the mentor acting as a role model, social support, tutor, and peer resource for the mentee. In a control group study the facilities using this program had significant increases in retention of both experienced and new assistants.

The next example of a successful orientation program was implemented in a Visiting Nurse Agency in Denver.[18] This program's essential components included (1) streamlining the orientation process and (2) improving communication among participants. Each new employee received a schedule of the time, place, and purpose of each phase of the orientation. Checklists noting each training phase were also provided so that new employees could ensure they were receiving all necessary information.

This orientation program also had a mentor system that provided a peer who accompanied the new home care assistant on the first day of work. As in the nursing home program, being a mentor enhanced status, and administration recognized the mentor for his or her experience and performance. Mentors were required to go through training to ensure consistency.

The last example of an effective orientation program used role-playing of difficult situations that required management of combative behavior, expressions of anger or fear, depression, or confusion.[19] Employees were expected to demonstrate skills, as well as pass a quiz on aging and attitudes toward caring for seniors. Results were discussed individually, and individualized programs were designed to strengthen skills under the supervision of the in-service coordinator, head nurse, or team leader. A year later, the nursing home had a 50% decrease in care assistant turnover. Surveys showed employees thought the behavior management exercises were especially helpful and gave credit to the thorough orientation program for their continued employment.

These facilities and agencies all reported significant improvements in turn-over rates. Additionally, some new employees reported increased pride in being a care assistant or in working for a particular organization. Many stated that they really liked the mentor system and felt an immediate sense of belonging and support. Other substantial additions to programming included developing content into writing for consistency and thoroughness, adding experiential exercises, providing one-to-one mentoring, implementing post-testing (whether paper and pencil or demonstration), developing individualized follow-up plans based on weaknesses identified in post-testing, and involving nursing staff in development and implementation.

Career Ladders

Career ladders are a response to care assistants' dissatisfaction with their "dead end" positions. They are structured programs with educational requirements, evaluation monitoring, and opportunities for reaching advanced levels of care provision. Upon meeting the criteria for advancement, assistants acquire new responsibilities and receive higher wages, as well as increased respect from peers and supervisors. Successful Career ladder programs combine three key elements: (1) an education component; (2) both empowerment and status advancements; and (3) improved salaries.

The following career ladders have evolved into national programs, purchased by and implemented in many nursing homes throughout the United States. The first program, Genesis, started in Massachusetts as a pilot project in 1987 and is currently used by over 50 facilities in 12 states.[20] This program consists of three rungs. The first rung for assistants is the Geriatric Nursing Assistant Specialist (GNAS). To be eligible, employees must work a minimum of 6 months and have above-average performance evaluations. They must then successfully complete six months of specified classes at local community colleges. Classes meet twice a week, and employees must take them on their own time. There are 6 modules, covering 100 hours and ranging from anatomy and physiology to performing senior assessments. Employees can miss no more than four classes per module in order to graduate; when the assistants comply with this rule, the nursing homes pay for the courses.

The second rung is Senior Nursing Assistant (SNA). SNAs prepare assignments, oversee other NAs, and hold NA meetings. Education consists of 30 hours of leadership training to facilitate adjustment to this new role. Classes cover motivation, conflict resolution, leadership styles, and communication. The third level is Senior Aide Coordinator (SAC).There is only one coordinator per facility. She or he serves as team leader for all care assistants. To be eligible, an assistant must have been at the first two levels for one year each, receive high performance evaluations, and demonstrate organizational, technical, and communication skills. The final step in this career ladder, offered to both NAs and LPNs, is to participate in a part-time flexible program to obtain an AS nursing degree. This allows employees to remain employed while pursuing educational goals. For the first year after graduation, retention levels are 98%, and they gradually drop to the high 80s after 4 years. Fifteen percent of participants went on to further formalized education.

INS CareWorks (of Integrated Health Services) is a career ladder program which has been implemented in nearly 300 facilities and has reduced turnover by 30 to 40%.[21] Its primary components are a 19-unit curriculum that covers key areas of assistants' work and a mentoring program that creates a support system for new staff. Two levels exist within the program. The first requires completion of a total of ten 3-hour training units. Assistants also work with many sources, including the MDS (Minimum Data Set) coordinator, to develop a care plan. Assistants also have a variety of hands-on experiences, from visualizing being admitted to a nursing home to wearing wet briefs. To be eligible to begin this first level, assistants must have no disciplinary actions against them, must be punctual, must have no appearance complaints, and must submit a 50-word essay describing why they want to be in the program. There is a cap-and-gown graduation ceremony with a reception dinner upon completion. Graduates receive a pay incentive and a new title, Caregiver I. To attain the Caregiver II level, nursing assistants work with an MDS coordinator in completing the MDS and RAPS (Resident Assessment Protocols) and developing responsive care plans and interventions. Assistants also get the opportunity to actually run a care-plan meeting. The curriculum at this level focuses on systems such as diabetes, arthritis, and pain management. The success of this career ladder program led registered nurses to seek their own program.

Apple Health Care, Inc. operates a chain of 21 nursing homes which have implemented a four-level career path for nursing assistants who do not wish to become nurses.[22] The program begins with a basic certification program for all nursing assistants. Then, three courses are offered over 4 months. Each of these courses is comprised sixteen hours of coursework designed to enhance their skills. These assistants earn quarterly bonuses for attainment of each level, and when all three courses are completed, annual earnings are increased by $1000. These certified nursing assistants (CNAs) are then eligible to participate in hiring and mentoring new aides and in developing more specialized caregiving skills. There are many other components of Apple Health Care's program, all aimed at making the nursing home more homelike and person-centered, with employees and seniors working together. Evaluations show employee turnover decreased an average of 30%, and these certified nursing assistants reported feeling more valued in the workplace. The administrators felt strongly that no single component was responsible for the improvement, but that the cumulative impact of all components led to a culture change. They also mentioned that nurses played a critical role in assistant job satisfaction. Nurses need training and development to succeed in their supervisory responsibilities, training they do not often receive in traditional nursing education.

Symbolic Tactics

Symbolic tactics are perhaps the easiest of all suggested strategies. Used alone they are usually ineffective and can be demoralizing. However, when used with other strategies, they reinforce a message of caring and concern. Following are some symbolic tactics found that target staff satisfaction and retention.[23, 24, 25, 26]

- Offering CNAs and nurses opportunities to attend offsite training programs, stressing the importance of networking with other healthcare professions.
- Providing new employees two new uniforms when they start, plus a new uniform every six months. If an employee leaves within six months, the cost of the uniforms is deducted from wages at the last paycheck.
- Making bulk food available to workers through an employee-run cooperative.
- Offering vans for employee carpools and for senior transportation.
- Contracting with landlords for an apartment building, offering timely payment for all units, in return for below-market-value rents. Offering employees a secure environment at significant monthly savings.
- Providing a paid-days-off plan that rewards workers and meets their needs. For example, in one facility, full-time employees received an annual deposit of paid-time-off days in a flex leave bank. These days included vacation time, all holidays, bereavement leave, and the first few days of sick time. At the end of the year, unused flex leave went into the employees' sick days' bank. This bank can build to 30 days, which takes employees to the beginning of short-term disability.
- Instead of offering service pins, letting employees choose their recognition awards from a gift catalog.
- Forming peer recognition committees for assistants and providing various forms of recognition.
- Creating a resource center, with computers available to staff on breaks, during lunch, and before and after work.

Exceptional responsiveness to clients and their families is another area requiring powerful symbolic tactics. These symbolic gestures not only send a message of caring and concern to clients and families, but also reinforce the importance of responsive caring. The following are some of the organization's tactics which are designed to support meeting and exceeding client expectations.[27]

- Providing small bouquets of flowers to hospice patients. These were donated by a local florist and delivered weekly by volunteers.
- Providing four free hours of services to families of clients who have passed away under the agency's care.
- Sending a staff member to the family's home during funeral services to help set up food and let people in and out.

- Sending birthday cards to clients and bringing birthday cakes to those without families.
- Developing a special fund for clients' non-medical requests (e.g., to help pay airfare for a son to come home to a dying client and to defray the cost of building a ramp at a client's home).
- Arranging with a local high school for volunteers to help clients with chores that the home care agency cannot perform.
- Sending thank-you cards to every discharged client.
- After three days of service, having an administrator call to see if services are meeting the client's expectations.

Just as with the previous list of tactics, none of these actions in itself will have much impact on clients or family members. However, the combination of these tactics when applied with other strategies reinforces the message of caring and responsiveness to seniors' concerns.

Training & Continuing Education

Often, first attempts to improve senior care focus on in-house education programs. Most programs evaluated positively influenced knowledge and attitudes; however, the most successful programs also influenced staff behaviors and seniors' outcomes. For example, some programs contributed to lowering turnover rates as well as decreasing use of restraints in nursing homes. Several programs garnered supplementary benefits, such as (a) increased staff opportunities to get to know supervisors; (b) decreased feelings of organizational isolation within; and (c) increased sense of organizational loyalty. [28, 29]

Successful training programs use of a variety of teaching methods, employ daily self-monitoring, and include nursing or supervisory involvement. Training courses should minimize didactic teaching, maximize interaction, and emphasize role-playing and other hands-on methods of building assistants' confidence and competence. Successful training uses principles of adult learning such as student participation, involving the mind as well as the emotions, and self-evaluations, which facilitate independence, creativity, and self-reliance.

An example of a home care training program that influenced assistants' knowledge, attitudes, and behaviors follows.[30] This education program was conducted in two home care agencies. The program's aim was to help assistants cope with emotional stress. The assistants received a total of 24 hours of in-service training, using demonstrations and on-going supervision, over the course of a year. At the year's end, a comparison of assistants in the in-service programs with those who did not participate revealed improved client-assistant relationships, increased assistant confidence, and increased ability to calm agitated clients. Furthermore, assistants who participated in the program did not personalize client anger as much as their control group peers did.

The next example of an effective in-service program focused on care assistants' behavior management skills.[31] The program started with a 5-hour curriculum taught by staff trainers for 3 weeks. Immediately following the in-services, behavioral skills were reinforced by working with RNs and LPNs on the job. Daily feedback was given to each assistant using a behavior management skills checklist for interactions with seniors. These skills checklists were also used for self-monitoring. To achieve eligibility for rewards, assistants had to have completed 80% of their daily self-monitoring forms, each of which took less than 5 minutes to fill out. The DON (Director of Nursing) also provided feedback in a monthly letter that summarized each assistant's overall performance for the month.

During the assistants' training, LPNs received supervisory-skills training. Each week supervisors completed a checklist similar to the assistants' for each enrolled assistant. This information was given to assistants to provide more on-the-job training. As a reward, all assistants who scored 80% performance or better had their names submitted to a weekly lottery. Each week, one name from each shift on each unit was drawn, and the winning individual received his or her choice from among four options: (1) a free lunch in the nursing home's cafeteria; (2) permission to arrive at work 30 minutes late; (3) permission to leave work 30 minutes early; or (4) one additional break during the day.

Observational data collected both prior to and after the training at monthly intervals revealed that assistants used the skills they had been taught. For example, assistants announced activities clearly and enthusiastically, made positive statements to the seniors, and gave seniors control over dates and times for their baths.

A unique in-service day for home care nurses, entitled "wellness day," focused on professional stress reduction.[32] Wellness was defined as "a sense of physical, mental, and spiritual well being that includes the ability to cope with challenges and live life to its fullest."[33] The day was held in a park, around a fire. Wellness workbooks were provided for each participant. The day included breakfast and guided imagery; yoga postures; a discussion of food and wellness; an exchange of low-fat, high-carbohydrate, and vegetarian recipes; and an affirmation hunt (prepared as an egg hunt). Stories using humor or imagery to help release stress were told, and music was played along with exercises designed to facilitate relaxing and healing. Finally, humor and music were used to poke fun at the trials and tribulations of assistants' jobs. Photos taken throughout the day were later arranged on a poster and displayed. The day provided nurses with a renewed sense of wellness in both their work and their lives. One nurse wrote in her evaluation, "My spirit is renewed. The day was such a gift! It has given me the energy and feeling of increased confidence in my ability to cope with the challenges of my work."[34]

Training must be implemented at all nursing levels in order to effect change. LEAP is a comprehensive program piloted in a nursing home and later replicated in three other facilities. (LEAP is an acronym corresponding to: *L*earning to use tools and resources for quality LTC, *E*mpowering caring and competence in self and others, *A*chieving commitment to work teams and the organization, and *P*roducing opportunities for growth and development.)[35] There are two modules of training. Module 1 is a six-week program for all nurse managers and charge nurses (RNs and LPNs) that is designed to develop leadership, gerontological expertise, and care teambuilding skills. Both didactic work and role-playing scenarios are part of the curriculum. Module 2 is a 14-hour workshop for NAs which focuses on career and skill development. The assistants' past performance evaluations, attendance history, letters of reference, formal applications, and interviews were all considered in determining who was accepted. Assistants who completed this program advanced to Level 2 and received a salary increase. Turnover rates for both nurses and assistants improved considerably in each facility. Fewer health deficiencies were found in all facilities, and nurses' and assistants' perceptions of their work empowerment, job satisfaction, and communication were significantly better.

Leadership, relationship, communication, and teambuilding skills are not "soft skills," Although they are often referred to as such. Rather, they are essential skills that significantly impact nursing staff turnover. Nursing staff education cannot continue to be viewed as an expense; high turnover rates are more costly. It was recommended that training to reduce deficiencies approach change as organizational learning and development.

One program that resulted in supervision training for nurses began with nursing assistants' brainstorming ways to eliminate the use of temporary staffing.[36] The program that developed in four facilities had four important parts: employee selection, orientation, scheduling, and supervision. Advertisements for direct-care jobs focused on the qualities of exemplary assistants, and all applicants were asked to follow experienced workers for two hours prior to being hired. The orientation process was redesigned to focus on core values instead of rules and regulations; scheduling was changed to self-scheduling, and a supervisory training program for nurses which addressed six key areas was created. Those key areas were (1) self awareness; (2) role acceptance; (3) teambuilding; (4) employee development and discipline; (5) solution orientation; and (6) personal organization. Within a year of implementing this multi-dimensional program, all four facilities involved had eliminated the use of temporary staff, and turnover rates in all facilities had decreased. Two received higher rankings in their senior care national survey (the other two had previously received the highest ranking).

In evaluating their program, the management learned several lessons. One of the most surprising was that most nurses did not think of nursing assistant supervision as their responsibility, and that many nurses who had started as nursing assistants thought of themselves as "just one of the workers."[37] The managers had to convince the nurses of their need for supervisory training by pointing out how much of the work for which nurses were held accountable was actually performed by nursing assistants.

Leadership and Managerial Skill Development

The leadership style of a nurse plays a pivotal role in both assistant satisfaction and client quality of care. Style includes a nurse's personal attitude, commitment, and interpersonal skills. Several studies found that when care assistants perceived their charge nurses as fair and competent, seniors' satisfaction increased.[38, 39, 40] Home care agency nurses have a similar, though not as strong, impact on staff and clients. One study found that nurses' motivation, communication, decision-making, and goal-setting correlated with homemakers' satisfaction, job involvement, and propensity to stay.[41]

The director of nurse's style profoundly impacts staff and clients. A study of 200 Australian nursing homes found that the leadership and managerial styles of nursing directors impacted nurses and assistants' team cohesiveness, general morale, and job satisfaction.[42] Based on these findings, the ten best caregiving homes were visited. Without exception, the nursing directors of high-performing homes were greatly respected by the nursing staff for their commitment and caring attitudes. This commitment was evidenced by the directors' dedication to high standards, enormous enthusiasm, and long working hours. Many of them were influential in professional organizations and senior advocacy groups. In all 10 nursing homes, the director of nursing was perceived to be the final authority and ultimate source of control in all matters relating to senior care.

The nursing director's style and managerial practices have been found to influence not only staff attitudes and behaviors but also seniors' quality of care. In another study, administrators completed a survey regarding the participatory decision-making style of their nursing directors.[43] Types of decisions nursing directors made (e.g., strategic, operational, and tactical versus senior care) and the scope of their decision participation (i.e., raising an issue, clarifying, generating alternative solutions, or deciding on solutions) were rated (and confirmed) by the DON. The outcomes of fractures, urinary tract infections, dehydration, and decubitus ulcers were also examined. Nursing director participation in decision making correlated with improvement in senior outcomes. In homes where nursing directors had the least decision making power, senior outcomes were poorest. Even after controlling for case mix, cost, facility size, and RN hours per senior, the participatory decision making style explained 20% of the variance in senior care outcomes.

Effectively developing nurses' leadership and managerial skills is not easy. Many leadership or managerial programs have been implemented in long-term care organizations, but few have provided valid evidence of changing nurses' behaviors enough to impact seniors. Both of the package programs presented at the beginning of this chapter found that one of the greatest contributors to decreasing assistants' turnover was supervisory training. Generally, these programs are expensive and must utilize many of the essential elements of effective in-services – individualized follow-up, minimal didactic teaching methods, and maximum interactive exercises. Additionally, the most effective programs coordinated training with managerial staff and care assistants.

One example of an effective leadership development program is entitled a "nursing management in-service and follow-up program" and was implemented in a 600-bed nursing home financed primarily by Medicaid payments in a metropolitan city.[44] Both the care assistants and the nurses were members of a local union, but each group had a different collective bargaining unit. The program began with a survey of nurses' attitudes and beliefs. The survey found that the nurses perceived the care assistants as a cohesive group with whom they felt powerless to work to improve care. The nurses also believed they had to be very accommodating toward assistants. For example, the nurses believed the assistants might slash their tires or complain to administrators about them if they asked assistants to perform more senior care. Furthermore, the nurses believed that minor disciplinary actions would not be backed up by supervisors.

Next, care assistants were interviewed using questions based on their findings from interviewing the nurses. The assistants knew that the nurses wanted them to function differently, that the nurses would not take disciplinary action, and that any disciplinary action would be insignificant and without administrative backing.

Following the interviews and surveys, nurses underwent a four-hour inservice / workshop and discussion session. The content included beginning principles of management and leadership, expert-based power, delegation, motivation, and discipline. At the same time, head nurses were encouraged to foster nurses' growth in managerial tasks and to delegate activities such as disciplining and performance appraisals to nurses. A second workshop was offered covering characteristics of cohesive groups, avoiding being manipulated, and initiating disciplinary actions.

Nurses then tried out several of these actions with the assistants. The nurses found that the expected behaviors of groups were more powerful motivators than were a manager's directions. The nurses got the assistants to agree to quality care values and actions. Gradually, as they asked assistants to perform care, the audible moaning decreased, and assistants took on the requested care tasks. Most significantly, the numbers of decubiti and incidents of restraint usage were decreased.

Primary Care and Permanent Assignments

Much of long-term care quality depends on holding nursing staff accountable to individual clients. With this in mind, several studies tested programs of primary care and permanent assignments for care assistants. In permanent assignment programs, each senior is assigned a care assistant and nurse who are responsible for him or her every day. This differs from the typical rotation model, in which client responsibilities are rotated among all care assistants. With permanent assignment, the nursing staff members know that they will be responsible for the same clients every day. Ideally, nursing staff can then implement special care and monitor outcomes more easily, while seniors can feel comfortable that their staff caregivers really know them. In primary care programs, a nurse or care assistant initiates care plans and manages them according to the client's preferences and health status. This primary care person is responsible for continual monitoring of health status and adjusting the care plan as necessary.

Permanent assignment programs have mixed outcomes. If the permanent assignment is one of several program interventions, the outcomes have been positive including increased feelings of personal control and choice, a decrease in disruptive behavior among seniors, and seniors' reports of feeling the quality of care was higher.[45, 46, 47] In one study, assistants reported that not only did they think they provided better care, but also that they were more aware of the seniors' needs.[48] A different study found that staff, seniors, and families preferred permanent staffing.[49] Families especially reported a greater sense of comfort in knowing the primary caregiver and the resulting improvement in continuity of care. Assistants reported a greater sense of responsibility and increased job satisfaction.

It must be noted, however, that permanent assignments by themselves do not consistently provide positive outcomes. One of the most carefully designed studies compared four nursing homes, two with permanent assignment, and two with rotating assignments. Seniors in the permanent assignment homes had significantly better personal appearance and hygiene, and nursing assistants reported greater job satisfaction. In the permanent assignment homes absenteeism was higher; however, staff retention was twice what it was in the rotating assignment homes.[50]

The first example of the use of the permanent assignment model is on one of two floors in two urban nursing homes in Illinois.[51] A great deal of planning took place to secure assistants' full cooperation. Assistants met with nursing supervisors many times to draw up fair and equitable lists of seniors before selecting their preferences. Although these meetings took much time, they laid the foundation for a successful transition and are now considered essential to making permanent assignments.

To evaluate the effectiveness of this model, permanent assignment charge nurses kept care records on each senior. Examples of items on care records were bed-bound seniors being turned every two hours or more frequently, and programs for bowel and bladder incontinence being followed. After three months, the permanently assigned assistants provided significantly better care. Permanent assignment reduced problem behaviors in all categories except complaining. For example, physical abuse went from 10 to 3% (control floors = 27 to 29%); verbal abuse went from 29 to 9% (control floors = 42 to 43%); resisting treatment went from 39 to 24% (control floors = 48 to 62%). Assistants' attitudes toward seniors improved slightly, while their job satisfaction decreased slightly. Positive staff outcomes were increased satisfaction with supervision and significant improvement in turnover rates, which fell from 16.9% to 4.8%, while control floors went from 17% to 19%.

After the 3-month trial, most assistants reported that they disliked the permanent assignment model and wanted to go back to the rotation model. The major source of dissatisfaction was that always working with the same seniors was boring and routine. One assistant said that when he woke up in the morning, he knew exactly what needed to be done for the seniors and when to do it. He said that he had to make his tasks last longer, or he would be done with all of his work an hour to an hour and a half earlier.[52] Another negative comment was that seniors became too demanding. For example, if an assistant was working with her senior, and the senior's roommate needed a glass of water, the roommate often would not let the assistant get it because the assistant was not assigned to him or her.[53] It is interesting that even though most aides did not like being permanently assigned, they believed that the model improved the quality of care. Seniors became more cooperative, more responsive to treatment, and experienced improved health.

The second example is of three nursing homes that implemented primary care at the assistant level.[54] Assistants got primary responsibility for special seniors. For example, it was up to them to figure out when to bathe. In most facilities the first six weeks were difficult, but, after this transitional period, assistants wanted the program to continue. Assistants' satisfaction with the model was high four years later. They noted that they could see their seniors' progress over time and their personal impact on seniors' lives. Seniors seemed to benefit too, as care related complaints from them and their families decreased significantly.

The last example involved three nursing homes which used a senior centered accountability model. This included (1) permanent assignment for assistants and (2) primary care nursing by case management nurses, which included seniors and assistants in care planning.[55]

An evaluation of this multi-pronged approach revealed mixed outcomes. The majority of nursing assistants were not happy with the permanent assignment component. Some said the seniors became too demanding and the concept got boring. The nurse supervisors of these care assistants were also ambivalent about permanent assignments. Those supervisors who wanted to know about problems greatly appreciated their new ability to identify them, but other supervisors disliked permanent assignment precisely because it made problem employees surface and obligated supervisors to take unpleasant actions. (Shortly after the program started, three assistants with considerable tenure were dismissed for abusing seniors.)

Regarding the primary care nursing by case management nurses, most assistants liked being included in the care planning process. Several assistants reported that they had started using care plans to direct their efforts. Nurses seemed to enjoy their role in planning care and the amount of control that seniors were given planning their own care. Seniors had different feelings. Some felt ganged up on by the staff. Others said the care planning gave them an opportunity to tell staff what they wanted and needed. Interestingly, most managers recognized that care plans had improved care but had difficulty supporting the concept because it decentralized authority so much.

In conclusion, primary care, senior centered accountability results in improvement for seniors and for nurses. Assistants' attitudes toward seniors and their control of choices were generally negative, but it was suggested that they could be influenced positively by in-service education programs. Permanent assignment resulted in greater control and satisfaction for seniors and less control and satisfaction for NAs.

Geriatric Specialist Nurses

Studies of advanced practice nurses, such as clinical nurse specialists and geriatric nurse practitioners, working in nursing homes have shown they can improve health outcomes without additional costs. Some health outcomes garnered from having advanced practice nurses in homes are fewer medication errors, fewer emergency room visits, more bowel and bladder control, and less use of restraints. Another significant outcome is a changed focus from custodial to rehabilitative care.[56]

A different approach to incorporating advanced practice nursing is to hire a hospital liaison nurse. One study used a liaison nurse to visit and consult with staff in eight nursing homes a minimum of once a month. The goal, to reduce seniors' emergency room visits and hospital readmissions, was achieved. The most common liaison recommendations were greater interdisciplinary collaboration, closer monitoring of lab work, and greater accuracy in fluid intake records.[57]

Home care agencies are starting to use advanced practice nurses as well. One agency saw the need for nurse specialists as their clients' hospital stays grew shorter and more high-technology services were necessary.[58] Nurse specialists in the areas of wounds, diabetes, cardiac rehabilitation, pulmonary care, and mental health were hired. These specialty nurses improved outcomes in seniors' health, in nurses' productivity, and in providers' growth. The agency had two methods of acquiring these nurse specialists: (1) providing specialty training to a seasoned home care nurses and (2) hiring a specialist while requiring her to acquire home care experience. Health outcomes included fewer medical complications, fewer readmissions, less frequent use of healthcare resources, speedier recovery, stabilized physical test results, and enhanced self-care skills for seniors. Outcomes among the nurses included keener assessments, clearer documentation, better technological skills, and more individualized client education. Of course, nurse specialists improved the home care agency's reputation, making accreditation easier to obtain, and increasing doctor referrals and managed-care contracts.

Basic Security—Wages, Hours, Benefits

The typical assistant is poorly paid and lacks basic benefits such as health insurance, paid vacation, and sick leave. If an assistant can earn more or receive benefits at a different facility or a fast-food place, then undoubtedly, she or he will consider changing jobs. While few studies have found pay to be the most crucial factor in assistants' decisions to quit, several surveys indicate that poor wages and benefits are among the top reasons assistants report for leaving their employers.[59] Some assistants report that low pay is running them out of the field they love and making their lives a constant struggle.

Disguised poor wages impact turnover just as much as obviously poor wages do. One study of four Illinois nursing homes with turnover rates ranging from 30% to 217% found that homes offering approximately the same wages and benefits had strikingly different turnover rates.[60] In the three high turnover homes, compensation policies differed from those in low turnover homes. High turnover homes paid their assistants for a 7.5-hour workday, rather than an 8-hour day. This decreased assistants' weekly earnings while keeping the hourly wage comparable to other homes. Surprisingly, in one home, assistants were not paid for their half-hour lunch but were expected to respond to calls for assistance during that time.[61]

Wage increases were frequently incorporated into programs with multiple components, but they were never the major focus. One program, Strategies to Reduce Turnover (SRT), made wage increases its foundation component.[62] SRT used Maslow's hierarchy of needs as a framework to organize its turnover reduction strategies. Physiological needs are the most basic, and in this program they were met via wage increases. All nursing assistants started at $9 an hour with yearly raises based on increases in the market and the cost of living. To provide for this increased wage, the number of staff members was decreased; all were cross-trained; and all nursing assistants, activity aides, and housekeepers (as well as nurses) were expected to help out at crucial times. Additionally, pay differences between frontline workers in dietary, recreation, and nursing were eliminated, with workers in the other departments cross-trained to perform assistants' work. Other components of SRT included addressing needs for belonging (through interdisciplinary decision making teams), feelings of self-worth, and self actualization. Prior to this program, the staff turnover rate was at 72%; in four years it had dropped to 17%, and was down to 10% in five years. Client satisfaction rates rose, while infection rates were significantly reduced. Best of all, the facility reported having to institute a waiting list for people who want to work there as nursing assistants.

Increase Nursing Staff

The preponderance of evidence from a number of studies using many measures of quality shows a positive relationship between numbers of nursing staff and quality of care. Considering the typical nursing staff levels in nursing homes, there is clearly a strong need to increase the overall numbers of nursing staff in nursing homes. The first landmark study in this area found that higher numbers of RN hours per client were associated with improved functional status, survival rates, and discharge rates of seniors to the community.[63] In a different study of 390 veterans discharged to 11 nursing homes, Barbara Braun found that RN hours were significantly related to veterans' mortality.[64] In other words, the more nurses in a facility, the less probability the veterans faced death.

Similarly, another study found that staffing ratios per seniors have a significant impact on seniors' health status and that staff mix (the number of staff assigned to severely disabled, moderately and mildly disabled seniors) is more important than overall numbers of staff.[65] Mortality within a year, having a bedsore, and functioning were tested for relationships with staffing FTEs (full time equivalents) per 100 seniors, adjusted for case mix. A higher RN ratio was associated with lower mortality rates. The authors calculated that an addition of half of an FTE RN (on average, about a 10-percent increase in RN staffing) would save about 3,000 lives annually.

It was also found that a higher intensity of LPN staffing improved seniors' functional status, although this impact was relatively small. Having more NAs had no impact on senior outcomes, at least not those measured in this study. Furthermore, it was found that low RN and LPN turnover was related to greater functional improvement among seniors. Taking nursing staff studies in a new direction, Zinn and her colleagues found that lower ratios of RN staff to seniors were associated with higher RN competitive wages.[66] Higher RN wages and fewer RNs were in turn associated with more frequent use of urinary catheters, physical restraints, tube feedings, and with seniors not routinely toileted. [67]

These data indicate the importance of RN staff to a nursing home. High quality facilities not only staff at higher levels than their low quality counterparts, they also staff at levels higher than national mean (0.42 compared to 0.34 hours per senior), while low-quality facilities staff at less than the national mean (.29 hours per senior, per day). A low quality facility would be nearly twice as likely to become a high quality facility if it increased its RN staff by 15 minutes per senior per day (or 3.3 RN FTEs per day per100 seniors).

The majority of studies in this chapter aimed to determine which managerial factors were most strongly related to turnover. While no single determining factor has emerged, a host of positive organizational factors have been found to significantly decrease nursing assistants' desire to quit. Supportive supervision, opportunities to express ideas, and opportunities for learning and growth are just some of them. Three seemingly unrelated variables—the number of beds, the number of beds per RN, and the number of beds per social service worker—were also correlated with turnover.

Conclusion

This chapter presents many successful and creative programs. Each approach addressed one or more of the nursing staff's or seniors' concerns. Although the majority focused on reducing staff turnover, in the process of reaching this goal most also addressed other areas of concern to seniors and assistants. Some programs concentrated on meeting seniors' needs for control and belonging, while others addressed assistants' need for respect and professional growth. Last, some programs addressed seniors' unspoken health and functional needs.

After considering program descriptions, a warning is in order. Implementing one or two of these strategies, no matter how wonderful they sound, will not accomplish the long-term goal of creating a caring, responsive *culture*. Quality care, both for staff and clients, is created by a combination of programs and necessarily varies from one organization to another. Furthermore, to be really successful, each organization needs to undertake participative planning in creating its own multi-dimensional programs. Additionally, constant monitoring of data regarding components and, most important, committed and responsive senior management, are needed. Without even one of these components, any success will be short-lived, as an exceptionally responsive culture cannot be superficially imposed.

The programs presented in this chapter represent fewer than one fourth of the strategies and programs reviewed in the literature. One reason for this is that many programs, while making valiant attempts, did not succeed. A second reason is that many program managers didn't measure success indicators. Without some evidence of success, funding is very difficult to attract, and programs are difficult or impossible to adjust appropriately. Another major reason there are so few successful programs is that they are expensive. A comprehensive approach is necessary, and this is quite costly. While it is relatively easy to obtain funding for one or two specific programs, establishing a more diverse, comprehensive package of programs is a formidable challenge. Last, new programs face several practical problems such as motivating senior management to invest in maintaining excitement and enthusiasm among the staff.

Quality, responsive care for seniors and staff is not an easily attained goal. Each weak area potentiates others. For example, high turnover reduces efficiency, imposes a financial burden, and creates an unpleasant work environment. This environment impacts seniors' lives, as addressing their health and emotional needs becomes more and more difficult. There is a compelling need to create a comprehensive approach to meeting and exceeding both seniors' and nursing staff's needs and expectations.

CR80

Discussion Questions

1.   Identify essential players in the Wellspring Model program and their roles.

2.   The Wellspring Model was duplicated in nursing homes other than the original eleven Wisconsin nursing homes. This duplication process forces each element of the program to be explicitly identified and described. Identify advantages and dangers of such explicit descriptions.

3.   In the Caring Touch program, it is said that the vocal tone and volume, level of listening, and degree to which the body relaxes are key. The aim of the Caring Touch program was to improve seniors' sense of caring. Three months after the implementation of this program, client outcomes were measured; however, more than a year later, nursing assistants were also interviewed about the program. What do you think is the most significant outcome of this program? What aspects of the program would make it particularly difficult to implement in other long-term care organizations?

4.   Often lessons can be drawn from carefully reviewing our "failures." The Outstanding Assistant of the Quarter program did not reach its intended goals. Identify lessons learned which will not be duplicated in the development of other new programs.

5.   Review the first seven client-focused programs. What common client outcomes were achieved? Compare the program components, identifying common ones.

6.   "Only one or two strategies cannot have a significant organizational impact. Multiple, appropriately chosen strategies, however, can have a significant impact." What programs are examples of these statements? What evidence supports these statements?

7.   Why can't one of the multi-strategy programs (e.g., the Wellspring Model or the Quality of Work Life home care program) be copied directly into other long-term care organizations with similar success?

8.   Several lists of symbolic tactics were provided; however, the warning was given that if they are used individually or in a piecemeal fashion they will probably be ineffective and could be demoralizing. Explain how this could happen.

9.   Five training programs were described which had positive outcomes on long-term care staff. After reviewing the programs, identify common program elements. How do you think these program elements influenced staff?

10.   Permanent assignments generally resulted in greater control and satisfaction for seniors and less control and satisfaction for frontline assistants. Provide suggestions to augment permanent assignments that would keep the client satisfaction high, but add staff satisfaction to it.

11.   Staff to client ratios, wages, guaranteed hours, and benefits are all primary job components. These program components are costly to improve. Can taking the plunge and improving staffing ratios, as well as wages, hours, and benefits guarantee better care? If not, what more is needed?

12.   Identify programs which despite their target had positive outcomes for both seniors and nursing staff. Compare these programs by human and fiscal resources. Which program do you favor and why?

References for Chapter 1

[1] Steil, L. and Bommelge, R. (2004). *Listening leaders: The ten golden rules to listen, lead, and succeed.* Edina: Beaver's Pond Press, Inc. p. 24

[2] He, W., Sengupta, M., Velkoff, V., and DeBarros, K. (2005). *U.S. Census Bureau, Current Population Reports, p23-209, 65+ in the United States: 2005*, U.S. Government Printing Office, Washington, D.C. p.13

[3] He, W., Sengupta, M., Velkoff, V., and DeBarros, K. (2005). *U.S. Census Bureau, Current Population Reports, p23-209, 65+ in the United States: 2005*, U.S. Government Printing Office, Washington, D.C. p.120

[4] He, W., Sengupta, M., Velkoff, V., and DeBarros, K. (2005). *U.S. Census Bureau, Current Population Reports, p23-209, 65+ in the United States: 2005*, U.S. Government Printing Office, Washington, D.C. p.135

[5] He, W., Sengupta, M., Velkoff, V., and DeBarros, K. (2005). *U.S. Census Bureau, Current Population Reports, p23-209, 65+ in the United States: 2005*, U.S. Government Printing Office, Washington, D.C. p.151

[6] He, W., Sengupta, M., Velkoff, V., and DeBarros, K. (2005). *U.S. Census Bureau, Current Population Reports, p23-209, 65+ in the United States: 2005*, U.S. Government Printing Office, Washington, D.C. p.100

[7] He, W., Sengupta, M., Velkoff, V., and DeBarros, K. (2005). *U.S. Census Bureau, Current Population Reports, p23-209, 65+ in the United States: 2005*, U.S. Government Printing Office, Washington, D.C. p.108

[8] He, W., Sengupta, M., Velkoff, V., and DeBarros, K. (2005). *U.S. Census Bureau, Current Population Reports, p23-209, 65+ in the United States: 2005*, U.S. Government Printing Office, Washington, D.C. p.101

[9] He, W., Sengupta, M., Velkoff, V., and DeBarros, K. (2005). *U.S. Census Bureau, Current Population Reports, p23-209, 65+ in the United States: 2005*, U.S. Government Printing Office, Washington, D.C. p.106

[10] He, W., Sengupta, M., Velkoff, V., and DeBarros, K. (2005). *U.S. Census Bureau, Current Population Reports, p23-209, 65+ in the United States: 2005*, U.S. Government Printing Office, Washington, D.C. p.83

[11] He, W., Sengupta, M., Velkoff, V., and DeBarros, K. (2005). *U.S. Census Bureau, Current Population Reports, p23-209, 65+ in the United States: 2005*, U.S. Government Printing Office, Washington, D.C. p.145

[12] He, W., Sengupta, M., Velkoff, V., and DeBarros, K. (2005). *U.S. Census Bureau, Current Population Reports, p23-209, 65+ in the United States: 2005*, U.S. Government Printing Office, Washington, D.C. p.165

[13] He, W., Sengupta, M., Velkoff, V., and DeBarros, K. (2005). *U.S. Census Bureau, Current Population Reports, p23-209, 65+ in the United States: 2005*, U.S. Government Printing Office, Washington, D.C. p.37

[14] He, W., Sengupta, M., Velkoff, V., and DeBarros, K. (2005). *U.S. Census Bureau, Current Population Reports, p23-209, 65+ in the United States: 2005*, U.S. Government Printing Office, Washington, D.C. p.1

[15] He, W., Sengupta, M., Velkoff, V., and DeBarros, K. (2005). *U.S. Census Bureau, Current Population Reports, p23-209, 65+ in the United States: 2005*, U.S. Government Printing Office, Washington, D.C. p.37

[16] Rowe, J. and Kahn, R. (1998). *Successful aging.* New York: The MacArthur Foundation Study Pantheon Books. pp.37-40

[17] He, W., Sengupta, M., Velkoff, V., and DeBarros, K. (2005). *U.S. Census Bureau, Current Population Reports, p23-209, 65+ in the United States: 2005*, U.S. Government Printing Office, Washington, D.C. p.54

[18] National Center for Chronic Disease Prevention and Health Programs, Centers for Disease Control and Prevention. Retrieved June 16, 2006 from the Centers for Disease Control and Prevention website at: http://www.cD.C.gov/nccdphp/programs/index.htm

[19] He, W., Sengupta, M., Velkoff, V., and DeBarros, K. (2005). *U.S. Census Bureau, Current Population Reports, p23-209, 65+ in the United States: 2005*, U.S. Government Printing Office, Washington, D.C. p.54

[20] He, W., Sengupta, M., Velkoff, V., and DeBarros, K. (2005). *U.S. Census Bureau, Current Population Reports, p23-209, 65+ in the United States: 2005*, U.S. Government Printing Office, Washington, D.C. p.59

[21] He, W., Sengupta, M., Velkoff, V., and DeBarros, K. (2005). *U.S. Census Bureau, Current Population Reports, p23-209, 65+ in the United States: 2005*, U.S. Government Printing Office, Washington, D.C. p.54

[22] He, W., Sengupta, M., Velkoff, V., and DeBarros, K. (2005). *U.S. Census Bureau, Current Population Reports, p23-209, 65+ in the United States: 2005*, U.S. Government Printing Office, Washington, D.C. p.57

[23] He, W., Sengupta, M., Velkoff, V., and DeBarros, K. (2005). *U.S. Census Bureau, Current Population Reports, p23-209, 65+ in the United States: 2005*, U.S. Government Printing Office, Washington, D.C. p.161

[24] He, W., Sengupta, M., Velkoff, V., and DeBarros, K. (2005). *U.S. Census Bureau, Current Population Reports, p23-209, 65+ in the United States: 2005*, U.S. Government Printing Office, Washington, D.C. p.66

[25] He, W., Sengupta, M., Velkoff, V., and DeBarros, K. (2005). *U.S. Census Bureau, Current Population Reports, p23-209, 65+ in the United States: 2005*, U.S. Government Printing Office, Washington, D.C. p.64

[26] Stone, R. (2000). *Long-Term Care for the Elderly with Disabilities: Current Policy, Emerging Trends, and Implications for the Twenty-First Century* Milbank Memorial Fund Policy Report p. 11

[27] Stone, R. (2000). *Long-Term Care for the Elderly with Disabilities: Current Policy, Emerging Trends, and Implications for the Twenty-First Century* Milbank Memorial Fund Policy Report p. 11

[28] National Council on Aging. (2000). *Senior Centers: Fact Sheet.* National Council on Aging, The National Institute of Senior Centers (NISC) Washington, D.C. Retrieved July 4, 2006 from the National Institute of Senior Centers website at: http://www.ncoa.org//content.cfm?sectionID=103&detail=1177

[29] National Council on Aging. (2000). *Senior Centers: Fact Sheet.* National Council on Aging, The National Institute of Senior Centers (NISC) Washington, D.C. Retrieved July 4, 2006 from the National Institute of Senior Centers website at: http://www.ncoa.org//content.cfm?sectionID=103&detail=1177

[30] National Council on Aging. (2000). *Constituent Groups: NISC: Accreditation.* National Council on Aging, The National Institute of Senior Centers (NISC) Washington, D.C. Retrieved July 4, 2006 from the National Institute of Senior Centers website at: http://www.ncoa.org/content.cfm?sectionID=131

[31] Center for Medicare and Medicaid. (2004). *Types of long-term-care and Medicare and home health care.* The Center for Medicare and Medicaid, Health and Human Services. Retrieved July 4, 2006 from the Center for Medicare and Medicaid, Health and Human Services website at:
http://www.medicare.gov/LongTermCare/Static/HomeCare.asp

[32] Center for Medicare and Medicaid. (2004). *Types of long-term-care and Medicare and home health care.* The Center for Medicare and Medicaid, Health and Human Services. Retrieved July 4, 2006 from the Center for Medicare and Medicaid, Health and Human Services website at:
http://www.medicare.gov/LongTermCare/Static/HomeCare.asp

[33] Day, T. (2006). *About long term care.* The National Care Planning Council. Retrieved July 4, 2006 from the National Care Planning Council website at: http://www.longtermcarelink.net

[34] American Association of Homes and Services for the Aging. (2006). *Services in housing.* The American Association of Homes and Services for the Aging. Retrieved July 4, 2006 from the American Association of Homes and Services for the Aging website at:
http://www.aahsa.org/advocacy/housing/services/default.asp

[35] He, W., Sengupta, M., Velkoff, V., and DeBarros, K. (2005). *U.S. Census Bureau, Current Population Reports, p23-209, 65+ in the United States: 2005,* U.S. Government Printing Office, Washington, D.C. p.162

[36] He, W., Sengupta, M., Velkoff, V., and DeBarros, K. (2005). *U.S. Census Bureau, Current Population Reports, p23-209, 65+ in the United States: 2005,* U.S. Government Printing Office, Washington, D.C. p.161

References for Chapter 2

[1] Roszak, T. (1998). *America the wise.* New York: Houghton Mifflin Company. p. 3

[2] American Association of Retired Persons' Policy and Strategy Group. (2004). *The state of America.* AARP, Washington, D.C.

[3] Bayer, A. and Harper, L. (2000). Fixing to Stay: A National Survey of Housing and Home Modification Issues. American Association of Retired Persons, Washington, D.C.

[4] Bayer A. and Harper, L. (2000). Fixing to Stay: A National Survey of Housing and Home Modification Issues. American Association of Retired Persons, Washington, D.C.

[5] Greenwald, M. and Associates, Inc. (2003). These Four Walls...Americans, 45+ Talk About Home and Community. Report of the American Association of Retired Persons, Washington, D.C.

[6] Krout, J., Wethington, E. (Editors). (2003). *Residential choices and experiences of older adults: Pathways to life quality.* New York: Springer Publishing Company, Inc.

[7] Belden, N., Russonello, J. & Steward, J. (2004) Caregiving in the U.S. The National Alliance for Caregiving in collaboration with the American Association of Retired Persons. Retrieved November 9, 2006 from the Caregiving in the U.S. website at: http://www.caregiving.org/data/04finalreport.pdf

[8] Gibson, M. (2003). Beyond 50.03: A Report to the Nation on Independent Living and Disability. American Association of Retired Persons Public Policy Institute, Washington, D.C., p. 8

[9] Gibson, M. (2003). Beyond 50.03: A Report to the Nation on Independent Living and Disability. American Association of Retired Persons Public Policy Institute, Washington, D.C., p. 30

[10] Gibson, M. (2003). Beyond 50.03: A Report to the Nation on Independent Living and Disability. American Association of Retired Persons Public Policy Institute, Washington, D.C., p. 7

[11] Roszak, T. (1998). *America the wise.* New York: Houghton Mifflin Company, p. 228

[12] Stricklin, M. (1993). Home care consumers speak out on quality. *Home Healthcare Nurse,* 11(6):13

[13] Stricklin, M. (1993). Home care consumers speak out on quality. *Home Healthcare Nurse,* 11(6):15

[14] Stricklin, M. (1993). Home care consumers speak out on quality. *Home Healthcare Nurse,* 11(6):10-17

[15] Forbes, D. (1996). Clarification of the constructs of satisfaction and dissatisfaction with home care. *Public Health Nursing,* 13(6):377-385

[16] Eutis, N. and Fischer, L. (1991). Relationships between home care clients and their workers: implications of quality of care. *Gerontologist,* 31(4):447

[17] Eutis, N. and Fischer, L. (1991). Relationships between home care clients and their workers: implications of quality of care. *Gerontologist,* 31(4):447

[18] Stricklin, M. (1993). Home care consumers speak out on quality. *Home Healthcare Nurse,* 11(6):16

[19] Glickman, L., Stocker, K., and Caro, F. (1997). Self-direction in home care for older people: a consumer's perspective. *Home Health Care Services Quarterly,* 16(1/2):41-54

[20] Degenholtz, H., Kane, R., and Kivnick, H. (1997). Care-related preferences and values of elderly community-based LTC consumers: can case managers learn what's important to clients? *The Gerontologist,* 37(6):767-776

[21] Siebert, J. (1996). Patient focus with an eye on the bottom line: using patient surveys for quality improvement. *Caring,* 15(10):26-37

[22] Siebert, J. (1996). Patient focus with an eye on the bottom line: using patient surveys for quality improvement. *Caring,* 15(10):26-37

[23] National Center for Assisted Living. Assisted Living: Independence, Choice and Dignity. (2001). Retrieved November 29, 2006 from http://www.ncal.org/about/alicd.pdf

[24] Zimmerman, S., et al. (2003). Assisted living and nursing homes: apples and oranges? *The Gerontologist,* 43(11):107-117.

[25] Krout, J. and Wethington, E. (Editors). (2003). *Residential choices and experiences of older adults: Pathways to life quality.* New York: Springer Publishing Company, Inc. pp. 43-45

[26] Hays, J., Galanos, A., Palmer, T., McQuoid, D., and Flint, E. (2001). Preference for place of death in a continuing care retirement community. *The Gerontologist,* 41(1):123-128

[27] O'Bryan, D., Clow, K., O'Bryan, J., and Kurtz, D. (1996). An empirical study of the influence of demographic variables on the choice criteria for assisted living facilities. *Health Marketing Quarterly,* 14(2):3-18

[28] Sherman, E., Venkatesan, M., and Chitnis, G. (1992). Customer satisfaction in the retirement living environment. *Journal of Ambulatory Care Marketing,* 5(1):17-26

[29] Krout, J. and Wethington, E. (Editors). (2003). *Residential choices and experiences of older adults: Pathways to life quality.* New York: Springer Publishing Company, Inc. pp. 27-46

[30] Shemwell, D. and Yavas, U. (1997). Congregate care facility selection: a conjoint approach. *Health Marketing Quarterly,* 14(4):109 - 120

[31] Sikorska, E. (1999). Organizational determinants of resident satisfaction with assisted living. *The Gerontologist,* 39(4):450-456

[32] Hawes, C. and Phillips, C. (2000). *High service or high privacy assisted living facilities, their residents and staff: Results from a national survey.* Miriam Rose Myers Research Institute.

[33] Wood, S. and Stephens, M. (2003). Vulnerability to elder abuse and neglect in assisted living facilities. *The Gerontologist,* 43(5):753-757

[34] Buelow, J. and Fee, F. (1999). Perceptions of care and satisfaction in assisted living facilities. *Health Marketing Quarterly,* 17(3):19

[35] Buelow, J. and Fee, F. (1999). Perceptions of care and satisfaction in assisted living facilities. *Health Marketing Quarterly,* 17(3):20

[36] Phillips, C., Munoz, Y., Sherman, M., Rose, M., Spector, W., and Hawes, C. (2003). Effects of facility characteristics on departures from assisted living: results from a national study. *The Gerontologist,* 43(5):690-695

[37] Zimmerman, S., et al. (2003). Assisted living and nursing homes: apples and oranges? *The Gerontologist, Special Issue,* 43(11):107-117

[38] Holder, E. and Frank, B. (1985). *A Consumer Perspective on Quality Care: The Residents' Point of View.* Report from National Citizens' Coalition for Nursing Home Reform, Washington D.C.

[39] Stein, S., Linn, M., and Stein, E. (1986). Patients' perceptions of nursing home stress related to quality of care. *The Gerontologist,* 26(4):424-430

[40] Holder, E. and Frank, B. (1985). *A Consumer Perspective on Quality Care: The Residents' Point of View.* National Citizens' Coalition for Nursing Home Reform, Washington D.C. p. II -12

[41] Stein, S., Linn, M., and Stein, E. (1987). Patients and staff assess social climate of different quality nursing homes. *Comprehensive Gerontology,* 1:41-46

[42] Noro, A. and Aro, S. (1997). Returning home from residential care: patient preferences and their determinants. *Aging and Society,* 17:305-321

[43] Stein, S., Linn, M., and Stein, E. (1986). Patients' perceptions of nursing home stress related to quality of care. *The Gerontologist,* 26(4):424-430

[44] Berdes, C. (1988). The modest proposal nursing home: dehumanizing characteristics of nursing homes in memoirs of nursing home residents. *The Journal of Applied Gerontology,* 6(4):372-388

[45] Stein, S., Linn, M., and Stein, E. (1987). Patients and staff assess social climate of different quality nursing homes. *Comprehensive Gerontology,* 1:41-46

[46] Joiner, C. and Freudiger, P. (1993). Male and female differences in nursing home adjustment and satisfaction. *Journal of Gerontological Social Work,* 20:3-4

[47] Noro, A. and Aro, S. (1997). Returning home from residential care: patient preferences and their determinants. *Aging and Society,* 17:305-321

[48] Holder, E. and Frank, B. (1985). *A Consumer Perspective on Quality Care: The Residents' Point of View.* National Citizens' Coalition for Nursing Home Reform, Washington D.C. pp. II 53-66

[49] Holder, E. and Frank, B. (1985). *A Consumer Perspective on Quality Care: The Residents' Point of View.* National Citizens' Coalition for Nursing Home Reform, Washington D.C. pp. II 13-23

[50] Stum, M. and Schmitz, K. (1990). *Quality Nursing Home Care: Family Roles and Perceptions.* Poster Session at Gerontological Society of America Annual Meeting. Boston, MA.

[51] Savishinsky, J. (1991). *The ends of time: Life and work in a nursing home.* New York: Bergin and Garvey. p. 169

[52] Savishinsky, J. (1991). *The Ends of time: Life and work in a nursing home.* New York: Bergin and Garvey. p. 75

[53] Berdes, C. (1988). The modest proposal nursing home: dehumanizing characteristics of nursing homes in memoirs of nursing home residents. *The Journal of Applied Gerontology 6(4)*:372-388

[54] Holder, E. and Frank, B. (1985). *A Consumer Perspective on Quality Care: The Residents' Point of View.* National Citizens' Coalition for Nursing Home Reform, Washington D.C. pp. II 24-34

[55] Buelow, J. and Fee, F. (1999). Perceptions of care and satisfaction in assisted living facilities. *Health Marketing Quarterly,* 1 (3) 2000. p.19

[56] Buelow, J. and Fee, F. (1999). Perceptions of care and satisfaction in assisted living facilities. *Health Marketing Quarterly,* 1 (3) 2000. p.20

[57] Buelow, J. and Fee, F. (1999). Perceptions of care and satisfaction in assisted living facilities. *Health Marketing Quarterly,* 1 (3) 2000. p.24

[58] Buelow, J. and Fee, F. (1999). Perceptions of care and satisfaction in assisted living facilities. *Health Marketing Quarterly,* 1 (3) 2000. p.20

References for Chapter 3

[1] Deutschman, M. (2000). What you hear when you listen to staff. *Nursing Homes Long Term Care Management,* 49(6):42

[2] U.S. General Accounting Office. (2001). Testimony by Scanlon, W. *Nursing Workforce: Recruitment and Retention of Nurses and Nurse Aides Is a Growing Concern.* GAO-01-750T. U.S. General Accounting Office: Washington, D.C.

[3] Yamada, Y. (2002). Profile of home care aides, nursing home aides, and hospital aides: historical changes and data recommendations. *The Gerontologist,* 42(2):199–206

[4] General Accounting Office. (2001).Testimony by William Scanlon, *Nursing Workforce: Recruitment and Retention of Nurses and Nurse Aides Is a Growing Concern.* GAO-01-750T. U.S. General Accounting Office: Washington, D.C.

[5] Brady, G., Case, A., Himmelstein, D., and Woolhandler, S. (2002). No care for the caregivers: declining health insurance coverage for health care personnel and their children, 1988-1998. *American Journal of Public Health,* 92(3):404-408

[6] Foner, N. (1994). Nursing home aides: saints or monsters? *The Gerontologist,* 34(2):p. 247

[7] Diamond, T. (1992). *Making gray gold: Narratives of nursing home care.* Chicago and London: The University of Chicago Press. p. 50

[8] Diamond, T. (1992). *Making gray gold: Narratives of nursing home care.* Chicago and London: The University of Chicago Press. p. 42

[9] Buelow, J. (2005). Author, shadowing frontline staff. January 2005.

[10] Herbert, B. (2002). The invisible women. The New York Times, September 12, 2002. Section A, Column 6; editorial desk, pg. 27

[11] Buelow, J. (2001). Author, shadowing frontline staff. December 1999.

[12] Feldman, P., Sapienza, A., and Kane, N. (1990). *Who cares for them? Workers in the home care industry.* Westport, CT: Greenwood Press. pp. 29-39

[13] Hartig, M. (1998). Expert nursing assistant care activities. *Western Journal of Nursing Research,*20(5):584-601

[14] Pinkerton, V. (2001). The value of home care assistance. *The Case Manager,* January/February, 12(1):43

[15] Hutchinson, R. (2001). *How do we fill New Hampshire's gap?* Paraprofessional Healthcare Institute and New Hampshire Community Loan Fund. p. 17

[16] Hartig, M. (1998). Expert nursing assistant care activities. *Western Journal of Nursing Research,*20(5):584-601, p. 594

[17] Hartig, M. (1998). Expert nursing assistant care activities. *Western Journal of Nursing Research,*20(5):584-601, p. 594

[18] Ebenstein, H. (1998). They were once like us: learning from home care workers who care for the elderly. *Journal of Gerontological Social Work,* 30(3/4):191-201

[19] Ebenstein, H. (1998). They were once like us: learning from home care workers who care for the elderly. *Journal of Gerontological Social Work,* 30(3/4):195

[20] Kahana, E. and Kiyak, H. (1984). Attitudes and behavior of staff in facilities for the aged. *Research on Aging,* 6 (4): 395-416

[21] Lidz, C., Fischer, L., and Arnold, R. (1992). *The erosion of autonomy in long term care.* New York: Oxford University Press, p. 41-56

[22] Bagshaw, M. and Adams, M. (1986). Nursing home nurses' attitudes, empathy, and ideological orientation. *International Journal of Aging and Human Development,* 22(3):235–246

[23] Schell, E. and Kayser-Jones, J. (1999). The effect of role-taking ability on caregiver-resident mealtime interaction. *Applied Nursing Research,* 12(1):38-44

[24] Schell, E. and Kayser-Jones, J. (1999). The effect of role-taking ability on caregiver-resident mealtime interaction. *Applied Nursing Research,* 12(1):40

[25] Schell, E. and Kayser-Jones, J. (1999). The effect of role-taking ability on caregiver-resident mealtime interaction. *Applied Nursing Research,* 12(1):42

[26] Bowers, B. and Becker, M. (1992). Nurse's aides in nursing homes: the relationship between organization and quality. *The Gerontologist,* 32(3):360-366

[27] Henderson, J., (1994) Bed, body, and soul: the job of the nursing home aide. *Generations,* 18(3):20-22

[28] Wagner, A. and Colling, J. (1993). Resistance to change: understanding the aides' point of view. *Journal of Long Term Care Administration,* 21(2):27-30

[29] Wagner, A. and Colling, J. (1993). Resistance to change: understanding the aides' point of view. *Journal of Long Term Care Administration,* 21(2):27-30

[30] Wagner, A. and Colling, J. (1993). Resistance to change: understanding the aides' point of view. *Journal of Long Term Care Administration,* 21(2):27-30

[31] Owen, B., Skalitsky-Staehler, K. (2003). Decreasing back stress in home care. *Home Healthcare Nurse,* 21(3):180–186

[32] Hartig, M. (1998). Expert nursing assistant care activities. *Western Journal of Nursing Research,*20(5):584-601

[33] Hartig, M. (1998). Expert nursing assistant care activities. *Western Journal of Nursing Research,*20(5):584-601

[34] Hartig, M. (1998). Expert nursing assistant care activities. *Western Journal of Nursing Research,*20(5):584-601, p. 595

[35] Hartig, M. (1998). Expert nursing assistant care activities. *Western Journal of Nursing Research,*20(5):584-601, p. 595

[36] Ebenstein, H. (1998). They were once like us: learning from home care workers who care for the elderly. *Journal of Gerontological Social Work,* 30(3/4):191-201

[37] Ebenstein, H. (1998). They were once like us: learning from home care workers who care for the elderly. *Journal of Gerontological Social Work,* 30(3/4):198

[38] Ebenstein, H. (1998). They were once like us: learning from home care workers who care for the elderly. *Journal of Gerontological Social Work,* 30(3/4):198

[39] Ebenstein, H. (1998). They were once like us: learning from home care workers who care for the elderly. *Journal of Gerontological Social Work,* 30(3/4):196

[40] Ebenstein, H. (1998). They were once like us: learning from home care workers who care for the elderly. *Journal of Gerontological Social Work,* 30(3/4):196

[41] Pillemer, K. and Moore, D. (1989). Abuse of patients in nursing homes: findings from a survey of staff. *Gerontologist,* 29(3):314-320

[42] Mercer, S., Heacock, P., and Beck, C. (1993). Nurse's aides in nursing homes: perceptions of training, work loads, racism, and abuse issues. *Journal of Gerontological Social Work,* 21(1/2):95-112

[43] Mercer, S., Heacock, P., and Beck, C. (1993). Nurse's aides in nursing homes: perceptions of training, work loads, racism, and abuse issues. *Journal of Gerontological Social Work,* 21(1/2):106

[44] Foner, N. (1994). Nursing home aides: saints or monsters? *The Gerontologist,* 34(2):248

[45] Foner N (1994). Nursing home aides: saints or monsters? *The Gerontologist,* 34(2):248

[46] Foner, N. (1994). Nursing home aides: saints or monsters? *The Gerontologist,* 34(2):249

[47] Carter R., Kooperman L., and Clare, D. (1988). Importance of perceived personal values in nursing home management. *The Journal of Long-Term Care Administration,* 16(2):10-13

[48] Holder, E. and Frank, B. (1985). *A Consumer Perspective on Quality Care: The Residents' Point of View.* National Citizens' Coalition for Nursing Home Reform, Washington D.C. pp. II 13-23

[49] Tellis-Nayak, V. and Tellis-Nayak, M. (1989). Quality of care and the burden of two cultures: when the world of the nurse's aide enters the world of the nursing home. *The Gerontologist,* 29 (3):307-313

[50] Brannon, D., et al. (1988). A job diagnostic survey of nursing home caregivers: implications for job design. *The Gerontologist,* 28(2):246-251

[51] Bye, M. and Iannone, J. (1987). Excellent care-givers (nursing assistants) of the elderly: what satisfies them about their work. *Nursing Homes & Senior Citizen Care,* 36(4):36-39

[52] Grieshaber, L., Parker, P., and Deering, J. (1995). Job satisfaction of nursing assistants in long-term care. *Health Care Supervisor,* 13(4):18-28

[53] Chichin, E. (1991a), The treatment of paraprofessional workers in the home. *Pride Institute Journal of Long Term Home Health Care,* 10(1):26-35

[54] Kennedy-Malone, L. (1996). Stay or stray phenomena. *Home Healthcare Nurse,* 14(2):103-107

[55] Diamond, T. (1992). *Making gray gold: Narratives of nursing home care.* Chicago: The University of Chicago Press. pp. 30-40

[56] Diamond, T. (1992). *Making gray gold: Narratives of nursing home care.* Chicago: The University of Chicago Press. p. 46

[57] Hutchinson, R. (2001). How Do We Fill New Hampshire's Gap? Paraprofessional Healthcare Institute and New Hampshire Community Loan Fund. p. 13

[58] Heiselman, T. and Noelker, L. (1991). Enhancing mutual respect among nursing assistants, residents, and residents' families. *The Gerontologist,* 31(4):552-555

[59] Pennington, K., Scott, J., and Magilvy, K. (2003). The role of certified nursing assistants in nursing homes. *Journal of Nursing Administration,* 33(11):578-584

[60] Bowers, B., Esmond, S., and Jacobson, N. (2000). The relationship between staffing and quality in long-term care facilities: exploring the views of nurse aides. *Journal of Nursing Care Quality,* 14(4):55-64

[61] Moyle, W., Skinner, J., Rowe, G., and Gork, C. (2003). Views of job satisfaction and dissatisfaction in Australian long-term care. *Journal of Clinical Nursing,* 12(2):168-176

[62] Chichin, E. (1992). Home care is where the heart is: the role of interpersonal relationships in paraprofessional home care. *Home Health Care Services Quarterly,* 13(1-2):161-177

[63] Kaye, L. (1986). Worker views of the intensity of affective expression during the delivery of home care services for the elderly. *Home Health Care Services Quarterly,* 7(2): 41-54

[64] Atkins, B., Meyer, A., and Smith, N. (1982). Personal care attendants: attitudes and factors contributing to job satisfaction. *Journal of Rehabilitation, July-September,* 48(3):20-24

[65] Donovan, R. (1989). Work stress and job satisfaction: a study of home care workers in New York City. *Home Health Care Services Quarterly,* 10(1/2):97-114

[66] American Health Care Association. (2003). Results of the 2002 AHCA Survey of Nursing Staff Vacancy and Turnover in Nursing Homes. Retrieved February 12, 2003 from the American Health Care Association website at: http://www.ahca.org/research/

[67] Schur, D., Noelker, L., Looman, W., Whitlatch, C., and Ejaz, F. (1998). 4 steps to more committed nursing assistants. *Balance,* 2(1):29-32

[68] U.S. Bureau of Labor Statistics. (2002). Employment Situation News Release, July 2002. Bureau of Labor Statistics, Washington D.C.

[69] Dunn, L., Rout, U., Carson, J., and Ritter, S. (1994). Occupational stress amongst care staff working in nursing homes: an empirical investigation. *Journal of Clinical Nursing,* 3(30):177-183

[70] Waxman, H., Carner, E., and Berkenstock, G. (1984). Job turnover and job satisfaction among nursing home aides. *The Gerontologist,* (24):503-509

[71] Grieshaber, L., Parker, P., and Deering, J. (1995). Job satisfaction of nursing assistants in long-term care. *Health Care Supervisor,* 13(4):18-28

[72] Mercer, S., Heacock, P., and Beck, C. (1993). Nurse's aides in nursing homes: perceptions of training, work loads, racism, and abuse issues. *Journal of Gerontological Social Work,* 21(1/2):95-112

[73] Mercer, S., Heacock, P., and Beck, C. (1993). Nurse's aides in nursing homes: perceptions of training, work loads, racism, and abuse issues. *Journal of Gerontological Social Work,* 21(1/2):110

[74] Case, B., Himmelstein, D., and Woolhandler, S. (2002). No care for the caregivers: declining health insurance coverage for health care personnel and their children, 1988-1998. *American Journal of Public Health,* 92(3):404-408

[75] Hutchinson, R. (2001). How Do We fill New Hampshire's Gap? Paraprofessional Healthcare Institute and New Hampshire Community Loan Fund, p. 22

[76] Hayashi, R., Gibson, J., and Weatherley, R. (1994). Working conditions in home care: a survey of Washington state's home care workers. *Home Health Care Services Quarterly,* 14(4):37-48

[77] Van Kleunen, A. and Wilner, M. (2000). Who will care for mother tomorrow? *Journal of Aging & Social Policy,* 11(2/3):1-11

[78] Hutchinson, R. (2001). How Do We Fill New Hampshire's Gap? Paraprofessional Healthcare Institute and New Hampshire Community Loan Fund, p. 18

[79] Case, B., Himmelstein, D., Woolhandler, S. (2002). No care for the caregivers: declining health insurance coverage for health care personnel and their children, 1988-1998. *American Journal of Public Health,* 92(3):407

[80] National Center for Assisted Living. Assisted living: independence, choice, and dignity. (2001). Retrieved November 29, 2006 from the National Center for Assisted Living website at: http://www.ncal.org/about/alicd.pdf

[81] Hutchinson, R. (2001). How Do We Fill New Hampshire's Gap? Paraprofessional Healthcare Institute and New Hampshire Community Loan Fund, p. 17

[82] Schur, D., Noelker, L., Looman, W., Whitlatch, C., and Ejaz, F. (1998). 4 steps to more committed nursing assistants. *Balance,* 2 (1):29-32

[83] Deutschman, M. (2000). What you hear when you listen to staff. *Nursing Homes Long Term Care Management,* 49(6):37-43

[84] Deutschman, M. (2000). What you hear when you listen to staff. *Nursing Homes Long Term Care Management,* 49(6):42

[85] Pennington, K., Scott, J., and Magilvy, K. (2003). The role of certified nursing assistants in nursing homes. *Journal of Nursing Administration,* 33(11):578-584

[86] Eaton, S. (2000). Beyond 'unloving care': linking human resource management and patient care quality in nursing homes. *International Journal of Human Resource Management,* 11(3):600

[87] Diamond, T. (1992). *Making gray gold: Narratives of nursing home care.* Chicago: The University of Chicago Press

[88] Grau, L., Chandler, B., Burton, B., and Kolditz, D. (1991). Institutional loyalty and job satisfaction among nurse aides in nursing homes. *Journal of Aging and Health,* 3(1):47-65

[89] Wagnild, G. (1988). A descriptive study of nurse's aide turnover in long term care facilities. *The Journal of Long Term Care Administration,* 16(1):19-23

[90] Schur, D., Noelker, L., Looman, W., Whitlatch, C., and Ejaz, F. (1998). 4 steps to more committed nursing assistants. *Balance,* 2(1):29-32

[91] Gaddy, T. and Bechtel, G. (1995). Nonlicensed employee turnover in a long-term care facility. *The Health Care Supervisor,* 13(4):54-60

[92] Kinder, C. (2003). Beyond wages: what do direct care workers want? *Best Practices,* 2(4):30

[93] Galloro, V. (2001). Call it a career. *Modern Healthcare,* 31(35):1-3

[94] Burke, G., Summers, J., and Thompson, T. (2001). Quality in long-term care: what we can learn from certified nursing assistants. *Annuals of Long-Term Care: Clinical Care and Aging,* 9(2):29-35

[95] Mercer, S., Heacock, P., Beck, C. (1993). Nurse's aides in nursing homes: perceptions of training, work loads, racism, and abuse issues. *Journal of Gerontological Social Work,* 21(1/2):95-112

[96] U.S. General Accounting Office. (2002). Nursing Homes Expenditures and Quality. GAO-01-944. U.S. General Accounting Office. Washington, D.C.

[97] Bowers, B., Esmond, S., Jacobson, N. (2000). The relationship between staffing and quality in long-term care facilities: exploring the views of nurse aides. *Journal of Nursing Care Quality,* 14(4):55-64

[98] Caudill, M. and Patrick, M. (1989). Nursing assistant turnover in nursing homes and need satisfaction. *Journal of Gerontological Nursing,* 15(6):24-30

[99] Gaddy, T. and Bechtel, G. (1995). Non-licensed employee turnover in a long-term care facility. *The Health Care Supervisor,* 13(4):54-60

[100] Wagnild, G. (1988). A descriptive study of nurse's aide turnover in long term care facilities. *The Journal of Long Term Care Administration,* 16(1):19-23

[101] Chichin, E. (1991a). The treatment of paraprofessional workers in the home. *Pride Institute Journal of Long Term Home Health Care,* 10(1):26-35

[102] Lusk, S. (1992). Violence experienced by nurses' aides in nursing homes. *Journal of American Association of Occupational Health Nurse,* 40(5):237-241

[103] Lusk, S. (1992). Violence experienced by nurses' aides in nursing homes. *Journal of American Association of Occupational Health Nurse,* 40(5):239

[104] Heiselman, T. and Noelker, L. (1991). Enhancing mutual respect among nursing assistants, residents, and residents' families. *The Gerontologist,* 31(4):552-555

[105] Van Kleunen, A., Wilner, M. (2000). Who will care for mother tomorrow? *Journal of Aging & Social Policy,* 11(2/3):1-10

[106] Galloro, V, (2001). Call it a career. *Modern Healthcare,* 31(35):1-3

[107] Paraprofessional Healthcare Institute. (2004). The right start. *Workforce Tools,* 1(2):1-7

[108] Atkins, B., Meyer, A., and Smith, N. (1982). Personal care attendants: attitudes and factors contributing to job satisfaction. *Journal of Rehabilitation, July-September* 48(3):20-24

[109] Caudill, M. and Patrick, M. (1991-2). Turnover among nursing assistants: why they leave and why they stay. *The Journal of Long-Term Care Administration,* 19(4):29-32

[110] deSavorgnani, A., Haring, R., and Davis, H. (1992). A survey of homecare aides: a personal and professional profile. *Caring,* 11(4):28-32

[111] Schur, D., Noelker, L., Looman, W., Whitlatch, C., and Ejaz, F. (1998). 4 steps to more committed nursing assistants. *Balance,* 2 (1):29-32

[112] Mercer, S., Heacock, P., and Beck, C. (1993). Nurse's aides in nursing homes: perceptions of training, work loads, racism, and abuse issues. *Journal of Gerontological Social Work,* 21(1/2):95-112

[113] Morgan, L. (1996). The quality of training for nursing assistants: evaluations of experienced workers. *Gerontology & Geriatrics Education,* 16(3):53-61

[114] Janz, M. (1992). Perception of knowledge: what administrators and assistants know. *Journal of Gerontological Nursing,* 18(8):7-12

[115] Kiyak, H., Namazi, K., and Kahana, E. (1997). Job commitment and turnover among women working in facilities serving older persons. *Research on Aging,* 19(2):223-246

[116] Hare, J. and Pratt, C. (1988). Burnout: differences between professional and paraprofessional nursing staff in acute care and long-term care health facilities. *The Journal of Applied Gerontology,* 7(1):60-72

[117] Novak, M. and Chappell, N. (1994). Nursing assistant burnout and the cognitively impaired elderly. *International Journal of Aging and Human Development,* 39(2):105-120

[118] Dawson, S. and Surpin, R. (2000). The home health aide: Scarce resource in a competitive marketplace. Bronx, New York: Paraprofessional Healthcare Institute

[119] Pillemer, K. (1996). Myths about nursing assistants. *Contemporary Long Term Care,* July:54-62

References for Chapter 4

[1] Hodges, L. (2001). Testimony of Linda Hodges, On Behalf of the College of Nursing University of Arkansas for Medical Sciences On the Nursing Shortage and Its Impact on American's Health Care Delivery System. American Association of Colleges of Nursing. Retrieved November 8, 2006 from the American Association of Colleges of Nursing website at: http://www.aacn.nche.edu/Government/Testimony/HodgesTestimony.htm

[2] Foreman, S. (2001). Optimal long-term care nurse-staffing levels. *Nursing Economics,* Jul/Aug, 19(4):164, 12p

[3] Braun, B. (1991). The effect of nursing home quality on patient outcomes. *Journal of American Geriatric Society,* 39:329-338

[4] Rantz, M., Azygart-Stauffacher, M., Popejoy, L., Mehr, D., Grando, V., Wipke-Tevis, D., Hicks, L., Conn, V., Porter, R., and Maas, M. (1999). The minimum data set: no longer just for clinical assessment. *Annals of Long-Term Care,* 7(9):354-360

[5] National Federation of Licensed Practical Nurses (2003). Retrieved November 8, 2006 from the National Federation of Licensed Practical Nurses website at: http://www.nflpn.org/index.html

[6] de Savorgnani, A., Haring, R., and Galloway, S. (1992). Caught in the middle: a profile of licensed practical nurses in home care. *Caring,* 11(9):12-13, 15-16

[7] Boeije, H., Nievaard AC, Casparie AF (1997) Coping strategies of enrolled nurses in nursing homes: Shifting between organizational imperatives and residents' needs. *International Journal of Nursing Studies 34(5):* 358-366

[8] Boeije H., Nievaard, A., and Casparie, A. (1997). Coping strategies of enrolled nurses in nursing homes: shifting between organizational imperatives and residents' needs. *International Journal of Nursing Studies,* 34(5):358-366

[9] Buelow, J. and Cruijssen, M. (2002). Long term care nurses speak out. *Nursing Homes Long Term Care Management,* 51(3):15-17

[10] Flores, S. (2000). Views from the American Assisted Living Nurses Association (AALNA). *Nursing Homes,* 49(3):50

[11] Wayne, A. (2004). Health care spending growth slows. *Provider,* 30(4):15-16

[12] Buelow, J. and Cruijssen, M. (2002). Long term care nurses speak out. *Nursing Homes Long Term Care Management,* 51(3):15-17

[13] Buelow, J. and Cruijssen, M. (2002). Long term care nurses speak out. *Nursing Homes Long Term Care Management,* 51(3):15-17

[14] Hedtcke C., MacQueen, L., and Carr, A. (1992). How do home health nurses spend their time? *Journal of Nursing Administration,* 22(1):18-22

[15] Ellefsen, B. (1998). Cooperation in community health nursing. *Nursing Leadership Forum,* 3(2):74-80

[16] Weaver, F., Perloff, L., Waters, T. (1998). Patients' and caregivers' transition from hospital to home: needs and recommendations. *Home Health Care Services Quarterly,* 17(3):27-48

[17] Weaver, F., Perloff, L., Waters, T. (1998). Patients' and caregivers' transition from hospital to home: needs and recommendations. *Home Health Care Services Quarterly,* 17(3):27-48

[18] Watson, R. (1991). Challenges in LTC nursing today. *Provider,* 17(9):14-18

[19] Fazzi Associates, Inc. (1998). From the consumer's perspective…what really matters. *CARING Magazine,* p. 61

[20] Hughes. K. and Marcantonio, R. (1993). Is there a difference? Nursing in proprietary and nonprofit nursing homes. *Journal of Gerontological Nursing,* 19(1): 28-34

[21] Shuster, G. and Cloonan, P. (1989). Nursing activities and reimbursement in clinical case management. *Home Healthcare Nurse,* 7(5):10-15

[22] Hughes, K. and Marcantonio, R. (1992). Practice patterns among home health, public health and hospital nurses. *Nursing and Health Care,* 13(10):532-536

[23] Hedtcke, C., MacQueen, L., and Carr, A. (1992). How do home health nurses spend their time? *Journal of Nursing Administration,* 22(1):18-22

[24] Hedtcke, C., MacQueen, L., and Carr, A. (1992). How do home health nurses spend their time? *Journal of Nursing Administration,* 22(1):18-22

[25] Wayne, K. (1999). Assisted living administrators need broad range of skills for 2000. *Balance,* 3(6):20-21

[26] Hawes, C., Phillips, C., Rose, M., Holan, S., and Sherman, M. (2003). A National Survey of Assisted Living Facilities. *The Gerontologist,* 43(6):875-882

[27] Tagliareni, E., Mengel, A., and Sherman, S. (1993). "Parallel worlds of nursing practice." Chapter in: Bruke, M. and Sherman, S. Ways of knowing and caring for older adults. National League for Nursing Press. p. 97

[28] Tagliareni, E., Mengel, A., and Sherman, S. (1993). "Parallel worlds of nursing practice." Chapter in: Bruke, M. and Sherman, S. Ways of knowing and caring for older adults. National League for Nursing Press. pp. 91-105

[29] Tagliareni, E., Mengel, A., and Sherman, S. (1993). "Parallel worlds of nursing practice." Chapter in: Bruke, M. and Sherman, S. Ways of knowing and caring for older adults. National League for Nursing Press. pp. 91-105

[30] Stulginsky, M. (1993). Nurses' home health experience, part II: the unique demands of home visits. *Nursing & Health Care,* 14(9):476-485

[31] Stulginsky, M. (1993). Nurses' home health experience, part II: the unique demands of home visits. *Nursing & Health Care,* 14(9):476-485

[32] Lidz, C., Fischer, L., and Arnold, R. (1992). *The erosion of autonomy in long term care.* New York: Oxford University Press. p. 54

[33] Davies, S. (1992). Consequences of the division of nursing labor for elderly patients in a continuing care setting. *Journal of Advanced Nursing,* 17(5):582-589

[34] Davies, S. (1992). Consequences of the division of nursing labor for elderly patients in a continuing care setting. *Journal of Advanced Nursing,* 17(5):582-589

[35] Lidz, C., Fischer, L., and Arnold, R. (1992). *The erosion of autonomy in long term care.* New York: Oxford University Press. p. 59

[36] Davies, S. (1992). Consequences of the division of nursing labor for elderly patients in a continuing care setting. *Journal of Advanced Nursing,* 17(5):582-589

[37] Tagliareni, E., Mengel, A., and Sherman, S. (1993). "Parallel worlds of nursing practice." Chapter in: Bruke, M. and Sherman, S. Ways of

knowing and caring for older adults. National League for Nursing
Press. pp. 91-105

[38] Tagliareni, E., Mengel, A., and Sherman, S. (1993). "Parallel worlds of
nursing practice." Chapter in: Bruke, M. and Sherman, S. Ways of
knowing and caring for older adults. National League for Nursing
Press. pp. 91-105

[39] Flores, S. (2000). Views from the American Assisted Living Nurses
Association (AALNA). *Nursing Homes,* 49(3).p.50

[40] Anderson, R. and McDaniel, Jr., R. (1992). The implication of environmental
turbulence for nursing-unit design in effective nursing homes. *Nursing
Economics,* 10(2):117-125

[41] Anderson, R. and McDaniel, Jr., R. (1999). R.N. participation in
organizational decision making and improvements in resident
outcomes. *Health Care Management Review,* 24(1):7-16

[42] Baldwin, D. and Price, S. (1994). Work excitement: the energizer for home
healthcare nursing. *Journal of Nursing Administration,* 24(9):37-42

[43] Baldwin, D. and Price, S. (1994). Work excitement: the energizer for home
healthcare nursing. *Journal of Nursing Administration,* 24(9):37-42

[44] Baldwin, D. and Price, S. (1994). Work excitement: the energizer for home
healthcare nursing. *Journal of Nursing Administration,* 24(9):37-42

[45] Kovach, C. and Krejci, J. (1998). Facilitating change in dementia care.
Journal of Nursing Administration, 28(5):17-27

[46] Kovach, C. and Krejci, J. (1998). Facilitating change in dementia care.
Journal of Nursing Administration, 28(5):17-27

[47] Turkel, M., Tappen, R., and Hall, R. (1999). Moments of excellence nurses'
response to role redesign in long-term care. *Journal of Gerontological
Nursing,* 25(1):7-12

[48] Turkel, M., Tappen, R., and Hall, R. (1999). Moments of excellence nurses'
response to role redesign in long-term care. *Journal of Gerontological
Nursing,* 25(1):7-12

[49] Turkel, M., Tappen, R., and Hall, R. (1999). Moments of excellence nurses'
response to role redesign in long-term care. *Journal of Gerontological
Nursing,* 25(1):7-12

[50] Turkel, M., Tappen, R., and Hall, R. (1999). Moments of excellence nurses' response to role redesign in long-term care. *Journal of Gerontological Nursing,* 25(1):7-12

[51] Chubon, S. (1991). An ethnographic study of job satisfaction among home care workers. *Caring,* 10(4): 52-54

[52] Chubon, S. (1991). An ethnographic study of job satisfaction among home care workers. *Caring,* 10(4): 52-54

[53] Turkel, M., Tappen, R., and Hall, R. (1999). Moments of excellence nurses' response to role redesign in long-term care. *Journal of Gerontological Nursing,* 25(1):7-12, (4):52-54

[54] Baldwin, D. and Price, S. (1994). Work excitement: the energizer for home healthcare nursing. *Journal of Nursing Administration,* 24(9):37-42

[55] Baldwin, D. and Price, S. (1994). Work excitement: the energizer for home healthcare nursing. *Journal of Nursing Administration,* 24(9):37-42

[56] Buelow, J. and Cruijssen, M. (2002). Long term care nurses speak out. *Nursing Homes Long Term Care Management,* 51(3):15-17

[57] Turkel, M., Tappen, R., and Hall, R. (1999). Moments of excellence nurses' response to role redesign in long-term care. *Journal of Gerontological Nursing,* 25(1):7-12

[58] Turkel, M., Tappen, R., and Hall, R. (1999). Moments of excellence nurses' response to role redesign in long-term care. *Journal of Gerontological Nursing,* 25(1):7-12

[59] Neal, L. (1999). The Neal theory: implications for practice and administration. *Home Healthcare Nurse,* 17(30):181-187

[60] Lynch, S. (1994). Job satisfaction of home health nurses. *Home Healthcare Nurse,* 12(5):21-28

[61] Chubon, S. (1991). An ethnographic study of job satisfaction among home care workers. *Caring,* 10(4):53

[62] Hoban, S. (2002). Long-Timers: Toby Lewis, RN: Reflections on long-term care nursing. *Nursing Homes Long Term Care Management,* 51(10):80-81

[63] Ellenbecker, C. and Warren, K. (1998). Nursing practice and patient care in a changing home healthcare environment. *Home Healthcare Nursing,* 16(8):531-539

[64] Ellenbecker, C. and Warren, K. (1998). Nursing practice and patient care in a changing home healthcare environment. *Home Healthcare Nursing,* 16(8):531-539

[65] Ellenbecker, C. and Warren, K. (1998). Nursing practice and patient care in a changing home healthcare environment. *Home Healthcare Nursing,* 16(8):531-539

[66] Mass, M., Buckwalter, K., and Specht, J (1996). "Nursing staff and quality of care in nursing homes." Chapter in: Institute of Medicine. Nursing staff in hospitals and nursing homes: Is it adequate? Committee on the adequacy of nurse staffing in hospitals and nursing homes. Washington, D.C. National Academy Press.

[67] Francis-Felsen, L., Coward, R., Hogan, T., Duncan, R., Hilker, M., and Horne, C. (1996). Factors influencing intentions of nursing personnel to leave employment in long-term care settings. *The Journal of Applied Gerontology,* 15(4):450-470

[68] Francis-Felsen, L., Coward, R., Hogan, T., Duncan, R., Hilker, M., and Horne, C. (1996). Factors influencing intentions of nursing personnel to leave employment in long-term care settings. *The Journal of Applied Gerontology,* 15(4):450-470

[69] Hood, J. and Smith, H. (1994). Quality of work life in home care. *Journal of Nursing Administration,* 24(1):40-47

[70] Curreri, C., Gilley, W., Faulk, L., and Swansburg, R. (1985). Job satisfaction: hospital-based RNs versus home health care RNs. *Nursing Forum,* 22(4):125-134

[71] Shuster, G. (1992). Job satisfaction among home healthcare nurses. *Home Healthcare Nurse,* 10(4):33-38

[72] Ellenbecker, C. and Warren, K. (1998). Nursing practice and patient care in a changing home healthcare environment. *Home Healthcare Nursing,* 16(8):531-539

[73] Moore, S. and Katz, B. (1996). Home health nurses: stress, self-esteem, social intimacy, and job satisfaction. *Home Healthcare Nurse,* 14(12):963-969

[74] Cohen-Mansfield, J. (1989). Sources of satisfaction and stress in nursing home caregivers: preliminary results. *Journal of Advanced Nursing,* 14:383-388

[75] Lynch, S. (1994). Job satisfaction of home health nurses. *Home Healthcare Nurse,* 12(5):21-28

[76] Beaulieu, R., Shamian, J., Donner, G., and Pringle, D. (1997). Empowerment and commitment of nurses in long-term care. *Nursing Economics,* 15(1):32-41

[77] Francis-Felsen, L., Coward, R., Hogan, T., Duncan, R., Hilker, M., and Horne, C. (1996). Factors influencing intentions of nursing personnel to leave employment in long-term care settings. *The Journal of Applied Gerontology,* 15(4):450-470

[78] Hood, J. and Smith, H. (1994). Quality of work life in home care. Journal of Nursing Administration, 24(1):40-47

[79] Beaulieu, R., Shamian, J., Donner, G., and Pringle, D. (1997). Empowerment and commitment of nurses in long-term care. *Nursing Economics,* 15(1):32-41

[80] Sorrentino, E. (1992). The effect of head nurse behaviors on nurse job satisfaction and performance. *The Journal of Long Term Care Administration, Hospital and Health Services Administration,* 37(1):103-113

[81] Buelow, J. and Cruijssen, M. (2002). Long term care nurses speak out. *Nursing Homes Long Term Care Management,* 51(3):16

[82] Buelow, J. and Cruijssen, M. (2002). Long term care nurses speak out. *Nursing Homes Long Term Care Management,* 51(3):16

[83] Buelow, J. and Cruijssen, M. (2002). Long term care nurses speak out. *Nursing Homes Long Term Care Management,* 51(3):15-17

[84] Mass, M., Buckwalter, K., and Specht, J (1996). "Nursing staff and quality of care in nursing homes." Chapter in: Institute of Medicine. Nursing staff in hospitals and nursing homes: Is it adequate? Committee on the adequacy of nurse staffing in hospitals and nursing homes. Washington, D.C. National Academy Press.

[85] Harrington, C. (1996). Nursing facility quality, staffing, and economic issues. Chapter in Nursing staff in hospitals and nursing homes: is it adequate? Washington, D.C. National Academy Press.

[86] Reed, J. and Morgan, D. (1999). Discharging older people from hospital to care homes: implications for nursing. *Journal of Advanced Nursing,* 29(4):819-825

[87] Rice, R. (1997). Home health care nurses report case load averages and daily visit frequencies: a national survey. *Geriatric Nursing,* 18(2):85-86

[88] Hilgendorf, P. (1996). Profile of the successful home health nurse case manager. *Nursing Management,* 27(10):32Q-32V

[89] Ellenbecker, C. and Warren, K. (1998). Nursing practice and patient care in a changing home healthcare environment. *Home Healthcare Nursing,* 16(8):534

[90] Ellenbecker, C. and Warren, K. (1998). Nursing practice and patient care in a changing home healthcare environment. *Home Healthcare Nursing,* 16(8):531-539

[91] Ellenbecker, C. and Warren, K. (1998). Nursing practice and patient care in a changing home healthcare environment. *Home Healthcare Nursing,* 16(8):531-539

[92] Boeije, H., Nievaard, A., and Casparie, A. (1997). Coping strategies of enrolled nurses in nursing homes: shifting between organizational imperatives and residents' needs. *International Journal of Nursing Studies,* 34(5):358-366

[93] Stulginsky, M. (1993). Nurses' home health experience, part I: the practice setting. *Nursing & Health Care,* 14 (8):402-407

[94] Baldwin, D. and Price, S. (1994). Work excitement: the energizer for home healthcare nursing. *Journal of Nursing Administration,* 24(9):37-42

[95] Hilgendorf, P. (1996). Profile of the successful home health nurse case manager. *Nursing Management,* 27(10):32Q-32V

[96] Buelow, J. and Cruijssen, M. (2002). Long term care nurses speak out. *Nursing Homes Long Term Care Management,* 51(3):15-17

[97] Buelow, J. and Cruijssen, M. (2002). Long term care nurses speak out. *Nursing Homes Long Term Care Management,* 51(3):15-17

[98] Ellenbecker, C. and Warren, K. (1998). Nursing practice and patient care in a changing home healthcare environment. *Home Healthcare Nursing,* 16(8):531-539

[99] Ellenbecker, C. and Warren, K. (1998). Nursing practice and patient care in a changing home healthcare environment. *Home Healthcare Nursing,* 16(8):531-539

[100] Hoban, S., (2002). Long-Timers: Toby Lewis, RN: Reflections on long-term care nursing. *Nursing Homes Long Term Care Management,* 51(10):80-81

[101] American Association of Homes and Services for the Aging. (2001). *Nursing home salary and benefits report.* Hospital & Healthcare Compensation Service, Oakland, N.J.

[102] Mass, M., Buckwalter, K., and Specht, J (1996). "Nursing staff and quality of care in nursing homes." Chapter in: Institute of Medicine. Nursing staff in hospitals and nursing homes: Is it adequate? Committee on the adequacy of nurse staffing in hospitals and nursing homes. Washington, D.C. National Academy Press.

[103] Harrington, C. (1996). "Nursing facility quality, staffing, and economic issues." Chapter in: Wunderlich, G., Sloan, F., and Davis, C. (Eds.). *Nursing staff in hospitals and nursing homes: is it adequate?* Committee on the Adequacy of Nurse Staffing in Hospitals and Nursing Homes. Washington, D.C. National Academy Press.

[104] Cadogan, M., Franzi, C., Osterweil, C., and Hill, R. (1999). Barriers to effective communication in skilled-nursing facilities: differences in perception between nurses and physicians. *Journal of the American Geriatrics Society,* 47(1):71-75

[105] Batteiger, T. (1995). Are home health care nurses happier? *Nursing Management,* 26(1):55-56

[106] Batteiger, T. (1995). Are home health care nurses happier? *Nursing Management,* 26(1):55-56

[107] Juhl, N., Dunkin, J., Stratton, T., Geller, J., and Ludtke, R. (1993). Job satisfaction of rural public and home health nurses. *Public Health Nursing,* 10(1):42-47

[108] Hare, J. and Pratt, C. (1988). Burnout: differences between professional and paraprofessional nursing staff in acute care and long-term care health facilities. *The Journal of Applied Gerontology,* 7(1):60

[109] Hare, J. and Pratt, C. (1988). Burnout: differences between professional and paraprofessional nursing staff in acute care and long-term care health facilities. *The Journal of Applied Gerontology,* 7(1):60-72

[110] Astrom, S., Nillson, B., Norberg, A., Sandman, P., and Winblad, B. (1991). Staff burnout in dementia: care-relations to empathy and attitudes. *International Journal of Nursing Studies,* 28(1):65-75

[111] Hare, J. and Pratt, C. (1988). Burnout: differences between professional and paraprofessional nursing staff in acute care and long-term care health facilities. *The Journal of Applied Gerontology,* 7(1):60-72

[112] Boeije, H., Nievaard, A., and Casparie, A. (1997). Coping strategies of enrolled nurses in nursing homes: Shifting between organizational imperatives and residents' needs. *International Journal of Nursing Studies,* 34(5):363

[113] Boeije, H., Nievaard, A., and Casparie, A. (1997). Coping strategies of enrolled nurses in nursing homes: Shifting between organizational imperatives and residents' needs. *International Journal of Nursing Studies,* 34(5):358-366

[114] Hinshaw, A. and Atwood, J. (1984). Nursing staff turnover, stress, and satisfaction: models, measures, and management. *Annual Review of Nursing Research 1*:133-53

[115] Seybolt, J. (1986). Dealing with premature employee turnover. *Journal of Nursing Administration,* 16(2):26-32

References for Chapter 5

[1] Epstein, S. (1995). Long-term care administration: from occupation to profession. *Nursing Homes,* 44(3):10-13

[2] Castle, N. (2001). Administrator turnover and quality of care in nursing homes. *The Gerontologist,* 41(6):757-767

[3] Kruzich, J., Clinton, J., and Kelber, S. (1992). Personal and environmental influences on nursing home satisfaction. *The Gerontologist,* 32(3):342-350

[4] Allen, J. (2003). *Nursing home administration, 4th Ed.* New York: Springer Publishing Company, Inc., p. 3-7

[5] National Association for Home Care and Hospice. (2005). *Professional certification of home care and hospice executives candidate information handbook.* Washington D.C.: National Association for Home Care and Hospice

[6] Brunk, D. (1998). Going pro. *Contemporary Longterm Care,* 21(5):62-67

[7] Lodge, M. (1987). Professional Education and Practice of Nurse Administrators / Directors of Nursing in Long-Term Care. Executive Summary American Nurses' Foundation, Inc. Kansas City, Missouri p. 1-48

[8] Scalzi, C. and Wilson, D. (1993). Analysis of job functions of top level nurse executives in acute, home, and long-term care: implications for education. *The Journal of Health Administration Education,* 11(1):57-65

[9] Scalzi, C. and Wilson, D. (1993). Analysis of job functions of top level nurse executives in acute, home, and long-term care: implications for education. *The Journal of Health Administration Education,* 11(1):57-65

[10] Roth, P. and Harrison, J. (1994). Ethical conflicts in long-term care: is legislation the answer? *Journal of Professional Nursing,* 10(5):271-277

[11] Singh, D., Shi, L., Samuels, M., and Amidon, R. (1997). How well trained are nursing home administrators? *Hospital & Health Services Administration,* 42(1):101-115

[12] Smith, H. and Chatfield, R. (1985). Managerial reports, profits, and quality of care: are they related? *The Journal of Long Term Care Administration,* 13(2):65-72

[13] Reid, W. and Coburn, A. (1996). Managerial responses to Medicaid prospective payment in the nursing home sector. *Hospital & Health Services Administration,* 41(3):283-296

[14] Peete, D. (1997). Administrators: transitioning from nursing homes to assisted living. *Nursing Homes,* 46(7):14-16

[15] Roth, P. and Harrison, J. (1994). Ethical conflicts in long-term care: is legislation the answer? *Journal of Professional Nursing,* 10(5):271-277

[16] Eliopoulos, C. (1992). Nursing administration manual for long term care facilities. Eau Claire WI: Health Education Network, LLC

[17] Todorovic, L., Fischer, M., and Hempler, J. (1997). A life care community from three perspectives. *Geriatric Nursing,* 18(5):223-226

[18] Todorovic, L., Fischer, M., and Hempler, J. (1997). A life care community from three perspectives. *Geriatric Nursing,* 18(5):223-226

[19] Boever, S. (1999). Helping your staff become more receptive to change. *Balance,* 3(3):10-12

[20] Kruzich, J., Clinton, J., and Kelber, S. (1992). Personal and environmental influences on nursing home satisfaction. *The Gerontologist,* 32(3):342-350

[21] Anderson, T. (1989). Priorities of expertise: what home care agencies look for in managers. *CARING,* Feb:49-59

[22] Vaughan-Wrobel, B. and Wittenauer, M. (1993). Management education: needs of nurse administrators in long-term care. *Journal of Gerontological Nursing,* 19(2):33-38

[23] Singh, D. (1997). *Nursing home administrators: Their influence on quality care.* New York & London: Garland Publishing, Inc. p. 89-94

[24] Todorovic, L., Fischer, M., and Hempler, J. (1997). A life care community from three perspectives. *Geriatric Nursing,* 18(5):223-226

[25] Scalzi, C. and Wilson, D. (1993). Analysis of job functions of top level nurse executives in acute, home, and long-term care: implications for education. *The Journal of Health Administration Education,* 11(1):57-65

[26] Roth, P. and Harrison, J. (1994). Ethical conflicts in long-term care: is legislation the answer? *Journal of Professional Nursing,* 10(5):271-277

[27] Singh, D. (1997). *Nursing home administrators: Their influence on quality care.* New York & London: Garland Publishing, Inc. p. 93

[28] Harrington, C., Mullan, J., Woodruff, L., Burger, S., Carrillo, H., and Bedney, B. (1999). Stakeholders' opinions regarding important measures of nursing home quality for consumers. *American Journal of Medical Quality,* 14(3):124-132

[29] Klaassen, P. (1998). Customer service trumps regulations. *Contemporary Long Term Care,* 21(4):92-93

[30] Harrington, C., Mullan, J., Woodruff, L., Burger, S., Carrillo, H., and Bedney, B. (1999). Stakeholders' opinions regarding important measures of nursing home quality for consumers. *American Journal of Medical Quality,* 14(3):129

[31] Harrington, C., Mullan, J., Woodruff, L., Burger, S., Carrillo, H., and Bedney, B. (1999). Stakeholders' opinions regarding important measures of nursing home quality for consumers. *American Journal of Medical Quality,* 14(3):124-132

[32] Simms, L., Pfoutz, S., and Price, S. (1986). Caring for older people: a challenge for nurse administrators. *Nursing Outlook,* 34(3):145-148

[33] Singh, D. and Schwab, R. (1998). Retention of administrators in nursing homes: what can management do? *The Gerontologist,* 38(3):362-369

[34] Singh, D. and Schwab, R. (1998). Retention of administrators in nursing homes: what can management do? *The Gerontologist,* 38(3):362-369

[35] Rubin, A. and Shuttlesworth, G. (1986). Job turnover among nursing home administrators: an exploratory study. *Journal of Long-Term Care Administrators,* 14(2):25-29

[36] Linder, R. (2001). Nursing home administrators: a vanishing profession? Press release from the National Association of Boards of Examiners of Long Term Care Administrators, Washington D.C.

[37] Rubin, A. and Shuttlesworth, G. (1986). Job turnover among nursing home administrators: an exploratory study. *Journal of Long-Term Care Administrators,* 14(2):25-29

[38] Singh, D. and Schwab, R. (1998). Retention of administrators in nursing homes: what can management do? *The Gerontologist,* 38(3):362-369

[39] Christensen, C. and Beaver, S. (1996). Correlation between administrator turnover and survey results. *The Journal of Long Term Care Administration,* 24(2):4-7

[40] Singh, D. and Schwab, R. (2000). Predicting turnover and retention in nursing home administrators: management and policy implications. *The Gerontologist,* 40(3):310

[41] Anderson, M., Slater, M., Aird, T., and Haslam, W. (1993). What to negotiate before accepting a DON position. *Geriatric Nursing,* 14(4):196-199

[42] Anderson, M., Slater, M., Aird, T., and Haslam, W. (1993). What to negotiate before accepting a DON position. *Geriatric Nursing,* 14(4):196-199

[43] Anderson, M., Slater, M., Aird, T., and Haslam, W. (1993). What to negotiate before accepting a DON position. *Geriatric Nursing,* 14(4):196-199

[44] Vaughan-Wrobel, B. and Wittenauer, M. (1993). Management education: needs of nurse administrators in long-term care. *Journal of Gerontological Nursing,* 19(2):33-38

[45] Wagner, L. and Vickery, K. (1999). The personal touch: The CEOs of two major long term care companies discuss their strategy, philosophy and resident focused approach to care. *Provider,* 25(6):30-43

[46] Peete, D. (1997). Administrators: transitioning from nursing homes to assisted living. *Nursing Homes,* 46(7):14-16

[47] Peete, D. (1997). Administrators: transitioning from nursing homes to assisted living. *Nursing Homes,* 46(7):14-16

[48] Pearson, A., Hocking, S., Mott, S., and Riggs, A. (1992). Management and leadership in Australian nursing homes. *Nursing Practice,* 5(2):24-28

[49] Kane, R. (1995). Improving the quality of long-term care. *Journal of the American Medical Association.* 273(17):1376-1380

[50] Kane, R., Frytak, J., and Eustis, N. (1997). Agency approaches to common quality problems in home care: a scenario study. *Home Health Care Services Quarterly,* 16(1/2):21-40

[51] Bilyeu, S. and Pagan, J. (2002). He said, she said: executive roundtable. *Contemporary Long Term Care,* 5(5):18–20

[52] Jones, P. (1988). The home care personnel shortage crisis. *CARING,* 7(5):6-9

[53] Jones, P. (1988). The home care personnel shortage crisis. *CARING,* 7(5):6-9

[54] Jones, P. (1988). The home care personnel shortage crisis. *CARING,* 7(5):6-9

[55] Jones, P. (1988). The home care personnel shortage crisis. *CARING,* 7(5):6-9

[56] Wayne, K. (1999). Assisted living administrators need broad range of skills for 2000. *Balance,* 3(6):20-21

[57] Wayne, K. (1999). Assisted living: new industry, new millennium. *Nursing Homes,* 48(12):68-69

[58] McGurk, J. (2000). Recruitment and Retention Strategies for Assisted Living Facilities. Assisted Living Federation of America Resources Executive Council, Alexandria, VA

[59] Kraus, E. (1974). Study reveals reasons for personnel turnover rates. *Modern Nursing Homes,* 32:48

[60] Krichbaum, K., Johnson, J., and Ryden, M. (1992). Educating nurses in leadership and management. *Geriatric Nursing,* 13(3):170-174

[61] Schleue-Warden, J. (1996) Members speak out on staffing! *The Director,* 4(4):126

[62] Schleue-Warden, J. (1996) Members speak out on staffing! *The Director,* 4(4):126

[63] Epstein, S. (1995). Long-term care administration: from occupation to profession. *Nursing Homes,* 44(3):10-13

[64] Pearson, A., Hocking, S., Mott, S., and Riggs, A. (1992). Management and leadership in Australian nursing homes. *Nursing Practice,* 5(2):24-28

[65] Riskin, C. and Zenas, C. (1989). Nursing education: management training needs unmet for LTC nurses. *Contemporary Long Term Care,* 49:49-50

[66] Vaughan-Wrobel, B. and Wittenauer, M. (1993). Management education: needs of nurse administrators in long-term care. *Journal of Gerontological Nursing,* 19(2):33-38

[67] Schmid, H. (1993). Nonprofit and for-profit home care in Israel: clients' assessments. *Journal of Aging & Social Policy,* 5(3):95-115

[68] Smith, H. and Chatfield, R. (1985). Managerial reports, profits, and quality of care: are they related? *The Journal of Long Term Care Administration,* 13(2): 65-72

[69] Davis, M., Freeman, J., and Kirby, E. (1998). Nursing home performance under case-mix reimbursement: responding to heavy-care incentives and market changes. *Health Services Research,* 33(4):815-834

[70] Davis, M., Freeman, J., and Kirby, E. (1998). Nursing home performance under case-mix reimbursement: responding to heavy-care incentives and market changes. *Health Services Research,* 33(4):815-834

[71] Smith, H., Fottler, M., and Saxberg, B. (1985). Does prospective payment encourage nursing home efficiency? *Evaluation & the Health Professions,* 8(2):209-221

[72] Will, K. and Nicovich, P. (2001). The best way to ensure long-term care's future: the professional education of administrators is vital to setting the stage for tomorrow's effective care delivery. *Balance,* 5(2):6-11

[73] Simms, L., Pfoutz, S., Price, S. (1986). Caring for older people: a challenge for nurse administrators. *Nursing Outlook,* 34(3):145-148

[74] Edwards, D. (2001). Training the greatest performers on earth. *Nursing Homes: Long Term Care Management,* 50(2):6-22

[75] Linder, R. (2001). Nursing Home Administrators: A Vanishing Profession? Press release from the National Association of Boards of Examiners of Long Term Care Administrators. Washington, D.C.

[76] Roth, P., Harrison, J. (1994). Ethical conflict in long-term care: is legislation the answer? *Journal of Professional Nursing,* 10(5):271-277

[77] Roth, P., Harrison, J. (1994). Ethical conflict in long-term care: is legislation the answer? *Journal of Professional Nursing,* 10(5):271-277

[78] Kane, R. and Wilson, K. (1993). Assisted living in the United States: a new paradigm for residential care for frail older persons. Retrieved November 8, 2006 from the *American Association of Retired Persons* website at: http://www.aarp.org/

[79] National Association for Homecare and Hospice. (1995). Profiles in Leadership. *Caring,* 14(10):26-38

[80] National Association for Homecare and Hospice. (1995). Profiles in Leadership. *Caring,* 14(10):26-38

References for Chapter 6

[1] Knox, R. and Upchurch, M. (1992). Values and nursing home life: how residents and caregivers compare. *The Journal of Long Term Care Administration,* Fall:8-10

[2] Knox, R. and Upchurch, M. (1992). Values and nursing home life: how residents and caregivers compare. *The Journal of Long Term Care Administration,* Fall:8-10

[3] Stein, S., Linn, M., and Stein, E. (1986). Patients' perceptions of nursing home stress related to quality of care. *The Gerontologist,* 26(4):424-430

[4] Adams, C., Johnson, J., and Moore, J. (1996). Patients' health problems: differences in perceptions between home health patients and nurses. *Home Healthcare Nurse,* 14(12):932-938

[5] Morrow-Howell, N., Proctor, E., and Rozario, P. (2001). How much is enough? Perspectives of care recipients and professionals on the sufficiency of in-home care. *Gerontologist,* 41(6):723-732

[6] Bagshaw, M. and Adams, M. (1986). Nursing home nurses' attitudes, empathy, and ideologic orientation. *International Journal of Aging and Human Development,* 22 (3):235-246

[7] Hare, J. and Pratt, C. (1988). Burnout: differences between professional and paraprofessional nursing staff in acute care and long term care health facilities. *The Journal of Applied Gerontology,* 7(1):60-72

References for Chapter 7

[1] McDonald, C. (1991-92). Career ladder: tool for recruitment, retention, and recognition. *The Journal of Long Term Care Administration,* 19(4):6

[2] Fazzi, R. (1991). Exceptional services, exceptional caring. *Caring,* 10(10):52-60

[3] Kehoe, M. and Van Heesch, B. (2003). Culture change in long term care: the Wellspring Model. *Journal of Social Word in Long Term Care,* 2(1/2):159-173

[4] Stone, R., Reinhard, S., Bowers, B., Zimmerman, D., Phillips, C., Hawes, C., Fielding, J., and Jacobson, N. (2003). Evaluation of the Wellspring Model for improving nursing home quality. Washington, D.C. Institute for the Future of Aging Services and American Association of Homes and Services for the Aging. pp. 1-43

[5] McDonald, M., McGuire, M., Sakauye, K., Schwartz, B., White, E., and Rosendahl, E. (1989). "Caring Touch: Training Nurse Aides to Enhance Quality of Life." Chapter 7 in: Day, J. and Berman, H. (Eds.). *Successful nurse aide management in nursing homes.* (1989). Westport, CT: Greenwood Publishing Group, Incorporated. pp.76-87

[6] Sinke, M. (1989). "Raising Productivity of Nurse Aides: An Incentive Program." Chapter 6 in: Day, J. and Berman, H. (Eds.). *Successful nurse aide management in nursing homes.* (1989). Westport, CT. Greenwood Publishing Group, Incorporated. pp. 66-75

[7] Ott, L. (1996). New design and management approach improves quality of life. *The Journal of Long Term Care Administration,* 24(1):52-54

[8] Ott, L. (1996). New design and management approach improves quality of life. *The Journal of Long Term Care Administration,* 24(1):53

[9] Ott, L. (1996). New design and management approach improves quality of life. *The Journal of Long Term Care Administration,* 24(1):54

[10] Christiansen, J. (2004). Northern Pines Community: culture change initiative. Retrieved July 10, 2006 from the Direct Care Clearinghouse website at: www.directcareclearinghouse.org/practices

[11] Doty, P. and Benjamin, M., et al. (1998). Comparing Client Directed and Agency Models for Providing Disability-Related Supportive Services at Home: Final Report. Los Angeles: University of California

[12] Wells, L. and Singer, C. (1988). Quality of life in institutions for the elderly: maximizing well-being. *Gerontologist,* April, 28(2):266-269

[13] Daehn, R. (2002). Get 'cart'-ed away. *Contemporary Long Term Care,* 25 (4):9-10

[14] Feldman, P. (1993). Work life improvements for home care workers: impact and feasibility. *The Gerontologist,* 33(1):47-54

[15] Stryker, R. (1982). The effect of managerial interventions on high personnel turnover in nursing homes. *The Journal of Long Term Administration,* 10(2):21-33

[16] Rajecki, R. (1990). Cut nursing aide turnover. *Contemporary Long Term Care,* 13(5):72-73

[17] Hegeman, C. (2003). Peer mentoring of nursing home CNAs: a way to create a culture of caring. *Journal of Social Work in Long-Term Care,* 2(1/2):183-196

[18] Ditson, L. (1994). Efforts to reduce homemaker/home health aide turnover in a home care agency. *Journal of Home Health Care Practice,* 6(4):33-44

[19] Tynan, C. and Witherell, J. (1984). Good orientation cuts turnover. *Geriatric Nursing,* 5(3):173-175

[20] McDonald, C. (1994). Recruitment, retention, and recognition of frontline workers in long term care. *Generations,* Fall 2004:41- 42

[21] Anders, K. (2001). How do you bait the hook? *Contemporary Long Term Care,* 24(3):24-28

[22] Misiorski, S. (2004). The pioneer network shares its approach to creating culture change in long term care. Retrieved June 16, 2006 from the Nursing Home Magazine website at: http://www.nursinghomesmagazine.com/Past_Issues.htm?ID=1518

[23] Anders, K. (2001). How do you bait the hook? *Contemporary Long Term Care,* 24(3):24-28

[24] Henry, G. (1993). Retaining CNAs in long term care. *Journal of Long Term Care Administration,* 21(2):18

[25] Packer-Tursman, J. (1996). Reversing the revolving door syndrome. *Provider,* 22(2):50-54

[26] Ditson, L. (1994). Efforts to reduce homemaker/home health aide turnover in a home care agency. *Journal of Home Health Care Practice,* 6(4):33-44

[27] Fazzi, R. (1991). Exceptional services, exceptional caring. *Caring,* 10(10):52-60

[28] Reagan, J. (1986). Managment of nurse's aides in long term care settings. *Journal of Long Term Care Administration,* 14(2):9-13

[29] Stevens, A., Burgio, L., Bailey, E., Burgio, K., Paul, P., Capilouto. E., Nicovish, P., and Hale, G. (1998). Teaching and maintaining behavior management skills with nursing assistants in a nursing home. *The Gerontologist,* 38(3):379-384

[30] Gibeau, J. (1993). Training paraprofessionals for psychiatric support. *Caring,* 12(4):36-42

[31] Stevens, A., Burgio, L., Bailey, E., Burgio, K., Paul, P., Capilouto, E., Nicovish, P., and Hale, G. (1998). Teaching and maintaining behavior management skills with nursing assistants in a nursing home. *The Gerontologist,* 38(3):379-384

[32] Tennant, K. (1997). Wellness for nurses, by nurses. *American Journal of Nursing,* 97(5):67-68

[33] Tennant, K. (1997). Wellness for nurses, by nurses. *American Journal of Nursing,* 97(5):67

[34] Tennant, K. (1997). Wellness for nurses, by nurses. *American Journal of Nursing,* 97(5):68

[35] Hollinger-Smith, L. (2003). It takes a village to retain quality nursing staff. *Nursing Homes Long Term Care Management,* May 03:52-54

[36] Davis, M. and S.Dawson, S. (2003). Pennsylvania's care gap: finding solutions to the direct care workforce crisis. *Paraprofessional Healthcare Institute,* p1-64

[37] Stevens, A., Burgio, L., Bailey, E., Burgio, K., Paul, P., Capilouto, E., Nicovish, P., and Hale, G. (1998). Teaching and maintaining behavior management skills with nursing assistants in a nursing home. *The Gerontologist,* 38(3):379-384

[38] Kruzich, J., Clinton, J., and Kelber, S. (1992). Personal and environmental influences on nursing home satisfaction. *Gerontologist,* 32(3):342-350

[39] Smith, H., Hood, J., and Piland, N. (1994). Leadership and quality of working life in home health care. *Home Health Care Services,* 14(4):3-22

[40] Pearson, A., Hocking, S., Mott, S., and Riggs, A. (1992). Management and leadership in Australian nursing homes. *Nursing Practice,* 5(2):24-28

[41] Buelow, J., Winburn, K., and J. Hutcherson, J. (1999). Job satisfaction of home care assistants related to managerial practices *Home Health Care Services Quarterly,* 17(4):59-71

[42] Pearson, A., Hocking, S., Mott, S., and Riggs, A. (1992). Management and leadership in Australian nursing homes. *Nursing Practice,* 5(2):24-28

[43] Anderson, R. and McDaniel, Jr., R. (1999). R.N. participation in organizational decision making and improvements in senior outcomes. *Health Care Management Review,* 24(1):7-16

[44] Burgio L, Fisher S, Fairchild K, Scilley D, Hardin M (2004) Quality of care in the nursing home: effects of staff assignment and work shift. *Gerontologist,* 44(3):368-377

[45] Burgio, L., Fisher, S., Fairchild, K., Scilley, D., and Hardin, M. (2004). Quality of care in the nursing home: effects of staff assignment and work shift. *Gerontologist,* 44(3):368-377

[46] Burgio, L., Engle, B., Hawking, A., McCormick, K., and Scheve, A. (1990). A descriptive analysis of nursing staff behaviors in a teaching nursing home: differences among NAs, LPNs, and RNs. *The Gerontologist,* 30(1):107-112

[47] Patchner, M. and Patchner, L. (1993). Essential staffing for improved nursing home care: the permanent assignment model. *Nursing Homes,* 42(5):37-39

[48] Burgio, L., Fisher, S., Fairchild, K., Scilley, D., and Hardin, M. (2004). Quality of care in the nursing home: effects of staff assignment and work shift. *Gerontologist,* 44(3):368-377

[49] Patchner, M. and Patchner, L. (1993). Essential staffing for improved nursing home care: the permanent assignment model. *Nursing Homes,* 42(5):37-39

[50] Burgio, L., Fisher, S., Fairchild, K., Scilley, D., and Hardin, M. (2004). Quality of care in the nursing home: effects of staff assignment and work shift. *Gerontologist,* 44(3):368-377

[51] Patchner, M. and Patchner. L. (1993). Essential staffing for improved nursing home care: the permanent assignment model. *Nursing Homes,* 42(5):37-39

[52] Patchner, M. and Patchner, L. (1993). Essential staffing for improved nursing home care: the permanent assignment model. *Nursing Homes,* 42(5):37-39

[53] Patchner, M. and Patchner, L. (1993). Essential staffing for improved nursing home care: the permanent assignment model. *Nursing Homes,* 42(5):37-39

[54] Hegland, A. (1994). DON of the year. *Contemporary Long Term Care,* 14(9):55, 57, 59

[55] Kaeser, L. (1989). "Nurse Aides and Quality of Life Nursing Care in Nursing Homes." Chapter 5 in: Day, J. and H. Berman. (1988). *Successful nurse aide management in nursing homes.* Phoenix: Oryx Press. p. 59-65

[56] Mezey, M., Greene, B., Bloom, H., Bonner, A., Bourbonniere, M., Bowers, B., Burl, J., Capezuti, E., Carter, D., Dimant, J., Jerro, S., Reinhard, S., and Ter Maat, M. (2005). Experts recommend strategies for strengthening the use of advanced practice nurses in nursing homes. *Journal of the American Geriatrics Society,* 53(10):1790-7

[57] Chappell H. Murrell, D. (1994). Nursing home patients: liaison nurse visits influence recidivism. *Journal of Gerontological Nursing,* May 20(5):33-36, 48

[58] Nemcek, M. and Egan, P. (1997). Specialty nursing improves home care. *CARING, June.* p. 12-18

[59] Holtz, G. (1982). Nurses' aides in nursing homes: why are they satisfied? *Journal of Gerontological Nursing,* 8(5):205-271

[60] Holtz, G. (1982). Nurses' aides in nursing homes: why are they satisfied? *Journal of Gerontological Nursing,* 8(5):205-271

[61] Baum, S. (1989). "Evaluation of Turnover Problem among Nursing Aides in Illinois Nursing Homes: Case Studies.: Chapter 2 in: Day, J. and H. Berman. (1988). *Successful nurse aide management in nursing homes.* Phoenix: Oryx Press. p.14-26.

[62] Garthe, K. (2004). Strategies to reduce turnover. Leelanau Memorial Health Center. Retrieved October 9, 2006 from the Direct Clearinghouse website at: www.directcareclearinghouse.org/practices

[63] Mass, M., Buckwalter, K., and Specht, J. (1996). "Nursing Staff and Quality of Care in Nursing Homes." Chapter in: Institute of Medicine. *Nursing staff in hospitals and nursing homes: Is it adequate?* Committee on the Adequacy of Nurse Staffing in Hospitals and Nursing Homes. Washington, D.C.: National Academy Press

[64] Braun, B. (1991). The effect of nursing home quality on patient outcomes. *Journal of American Geriatric Society*, 39: 329-338

[65] Spector, W. and Takada, H. (1991). Characteristics of nursing homes that affect resident outcomes. *Journal of Aging and Health*, 3(4): 427-454

[66] Zinn, J. (1993). The influence of nurse wage differentials on nursing home staffing and senior care decisions. *The Gerontologist*, 33(6):721-729

[67] Mass, M., Buckwalter, K., and Specht, J. (1996). "Nursing Staff and Quality of Care in Nursing Homes." Chapter in: Institute of Medicine. *Nursing staff in hospitals and nursing homes: Is it adequate?* Committee on the Adequacy of Nurse Staffing in Hospitals and Nursing Homes, Washington, D.C.: National Academy Press

Index

Index

About the Author

Janet Buelow, PhD, an Associate Professor of Health Services Administration, has personally fulfilled many of the roles described in this book. Beginning in 1974, she worked as a nursing assistant in several different nursing homes. She then worked as a nurse and as an administrator in nursing homes, rehabilitation hospital units, and public health departments. Since 1985, her research has focused on management practices and their impact on aging clients and nursing staff in long-term care facilities. Her research has been conducted in the long-term care settings of nursing homes, home care agencies, respite care centers, assisted-living facilities, and adult day care centers in highly urbanized, metropolitan areas and rural locations. The research has involved interviewing clients as well as frontline workers and nurses.

Dr. Buelow's current studies now include comparisons of long-term care managers' perspectives internationally and the facilitation of interdisciplinary education, crossing both business and medical paradigms. Currently, Dr. Buelow is at the University of South Dakota teaching in the Health Services Administration division and coordinating international programs for the School of Business. She teaches healthcare systems courses as well as long-term care seminars.

CR